9780397502806
AF544834

Cutaneous Lesions of the Lower Extremities

Cutaneous Lesions of the Lower Extremities

M. H. Samitz, M.D., M.Sc. (Med.)

Professor of Dermatology and Director of Graduate Dermatology, School of Medicine, University of Pennsylvania; Chief, Department of Dermatology, Graduate Hospital, University of Pennsylvania; Consultant and Professor of Dermatology, Pennsylvania College of Podiatric Medicine.

Alan S. Dana, Jr., M.D.

Associate in Dermatology, School of Medicine, University of Pennsylvania; Associate Dermatologist-Syphilologist, Graduate Hospital, University of Pennsylvania.

135 Illustrations in color

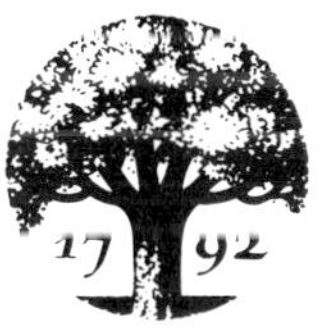

J. B. Lippincott Company

Philadelphia · Toronto

Distributed in Great Britain by
Blackwell Scientific Publications, Oxford and Edinburgh

Library of Congress Catalog Card Number 75-152141

Printed in the United States of America

3 2 1

Dedicated to

Our Residents and Students Who Have Made the Learning and the Teaching of Dermatology an Exciting Experience

Preface

Cutaneous disorders that show a predilection for the lower extremities are the subject of this text.

Lesions of the lower extremity are a significant diagnostic and therapeutic challenge not only to the general practitioner, but also to the internist, surgeon and dermatologist. It is hoped that this book will be useful in the teaching of dermatology in schools of podiatry, and practical information for the podiatric practitioner has also been emphasized.

Although the diagnostic importance of the regional localization of lesions can be exaggerated, there is often great significance in the specialized patterns of their distribution. This might involve cutaneous lesions that are the sole expression of disease—such as tinea pedis, which reflects purely local factors such as moisture, heat and maceration—or those cutaneous lesions that reflect a systemic disease affecting various organ systems, such as ulcers in hematopoietic disease or necrobiosis lipoidica diabeticorum seen with diabetes.

Topics have been selected on the basis of their importance in the clinical practice of the internist and dermatologist. New data on physiologic and biochemical properties that clarify skin function in health and disease are discussed, and clinical applications are emphasized.

The material is based on experience in our offices and in the dermatology clinics of the Hospital of the University of Pennsylvania and the Graduate Hospital of the University of Pennsylvania. Some ideas have been expressed by others; the selected bibliographies indicate the sources of this information.

Acknowledgments

We are very grateful to the members of our staff—Dr. Fillmore K. Bagatell, Dr. Charles L. Heaton, Dr. Marvin Greenberg, Dr. Richard R. Marples, and Dr. Jack Weiner—for their extremely helpful contributions with individual sections, and to our residents and graduate students who have given us valuable assistance in many ways. We wish to express our appreciation to Dr. Albert M. Kligman who read the entire manuscript and offered invaluable constructive criticisms.

We are indebted to John K. Abely, publisher, The Yorke Medical Group, for permission to reprint and reproduce material adapted from our series of four articles (pigmented purpuric eruptions, nodose lesions, ulcers and necrotizing vasculitides) originally published in *Cutis*, September-December, 1966; copyright, The Reuben H. Donnelley Corporation, and to Robert R. Kierland, M.D., Chief Editor, *Archives of Dermatology* for permission to reprint sections of our paper "*The hunting reaction,*" *99:*441, 1969 and to reproduce the illustration in "*Leg ulcers in Mediterranean anemia,*" *90:*567, 1964, and the illustration in "*Eccrine poroma,*" *98*:162, 1968.

We wish to express our thanks, also, to the staff and students of the Pennsylvania College of Podiatric Medicine for their cooperation and stimulation.

Over ninety percent of the illustrations are photographs of patients treated by the senior author over the past thirty years. Dr. Jack Weiner graciously permitted use of photographs from his collection, Dr. G. Ted Anderson provided the photographs in chapter 9, Immersion Injuries, and Dr. Samuel L. Moschella, Dr. Ira H. Rex, Jr., Dr. L. F. Fenster and Dr. William Heiss permitted the use of individual photographs. The placement of the color plates in proximity to related text was made possible by a grant from Schering Laboratories, Kenilworth, New Jersey.

M. H. Samitz, M. D.
Alan S. Dana, Jr., M. D.

Contents

1

Introduction

LOCALIZATION OF LESIONS ON THE LOWER EXTREMITIES

The distribution of skin diseases is interesting as well as puzzling. Knowledge of sites of predilection will frequently guide the clinician toward a diagnosis. Causes of the localization of skin diseases on the lower extremities are known in certain instances, such as contact dermatitis of the feet, monilial and dermatophyte infections, ulcers in association with incompetent veins or with diabetes, sweating disorders from wearing apparel and warm water immersion foot.

Many congenital abnormalities of the legs probably begin before the eighth week of in-utero life, since even the soles are grossly recognizable at that time. The cause of supernumerary digits, agenesis of digits and twinning of limbs, represent embryonic damage of unknown origin.

The development of callosities, warts and corns in areas of pressure is in part related to the excessive weight placed on a small skin area or to mechanical factors.

Abnormal constituents of the blood may result in a lesion occurring in the lower extremities because of the state of the local vasculature. Thus, the abnormal red cell in sickle cell anemia may be exposed to a more sluggish circulation in the legs, give up more oxygen and change its shape, to the extent that it becomes a cell that will not move as readily through the vessels. The blood vessel becomes occluded and the skin becomes devitalized and ulcerates. Macroglobulins may tend to aggregate in the same stagnated circumstances and cause tissue necrosis and ulceration. Cold may cause excessive amounts of cryoglobulins and cryofibrinogens to precipitate and produce devitalization of skin.

Damage to nerves from such disorders as syringomyelia, diabetes mellitus, leprosy, poliomyelitis and mercury hypersensitivity may cause insensitive limbs that are damaged and deformed by trauma. The feet and legs endure more insults than any other part of the body. Therefore, traumatic ulcers, foreign body granulomas, insect bites, cuts and infections may be more common on the legs. The interdigital spaces of some toes, such as the third and fourth interspaces, are relatively narrowed, allowing the skin to become macerated, and increasing the tendency to bacterial, dermatophyte and monilial infections.

Knowledge is inadequate to explain the localization of many skin problems ranging from rare heritable diseases such as Mal de Meleda and keratoderma palmaris et plantaris to acquired disorders such as pustular psoriasis, nodose lesions, necrotizing vasculitides and pigmented purpuric eruptions. It is possible that tissue activity in the lower extremities is programmed to behave different than it does in other parts of the body.

One must differentiate those cutaneous lesions which are strictly dermatologic entities from those which are the counterparts of lesions in internal organs. A simple classification may be used.

I. Heritable
  A. Genetic conditions in which the biochemical defect is still unknown. (e.g., epidermolysis bullosa, ichthyosis, Mal de Meleda, keratoderma palmaris et plantaris).
  B. Genetically determined diseases (inborn errors of metabolism).

II. Acquired
  A. Diseases due to external causes such as impetigo, contact dermatitis, dermatophytosis.
  B. Diseases due to internal causes.
    1. The skin lesion appears first and systemic involvement develops later (e.g., necrobiosis lipoidica diabeticorum with diabetes, scleroderma preceding systemic sclerosis).
    2. The skin lesion is secondary to the systemic disease (e.g., pyoderma gangrenosum with ulcerative colitis, leg ulcers due to hypertension, sickle cell anemia or diabetes, vesicles on the feet in hand, foot and mouth viral disease).
  C. Diseases limited to skin: strictly dermatologic entities of known and unknown origin (e.g., psoriasis, lichen planus, x-ray dermatitis).

It is essential for one to have a reasonable knowledge of:

1. The anatomy of the skin.

2. The relationship between structure and function.

3. The biochemical factors and physiologic alterations which play a role in causing the pathologic picture.

HUMAN SKIN

An understanding of human skin is incomplete without knowledge of skin functions in lower animals. The morphology and physiology of human skin is the outcome of a long period of phylogenetic development. None of the varied adaptive changes, such as the modification of the papillae of pads which is unique in different bird species, was necessary for man and therefore is not present in the human foot. The comparison of footpads in nonhuman primates with soles in man is pertinent. When man assumed the upright stance, a great burden was placed on the lower extremity. The soles of the feet helped meet this work load by presenting a thickened, tough stratum corneum.

Human skin totals about ten pounds of weight for the average-sized man, about seven pounds for the average woman. Estimates of the area of the human skin cover a wide range, up to 15,000 square inches — roughly the size of a nine-by-twelve rug. It is a complex, flexible, fibrous structure that encases all the living tissues and organs of the body. It is the most accessible tissue of the body and may serve as an excellent model for multidisciplinary research.

The skin is divided into three layers: epidermis, dermis (corium) and hypodermis (fatty layer).

EPIDERMIS

The epidermis has a thickness approximately equal to a sheet of paper. Most of it does not exceed 0.2 mm., although it is much thicker in the palms and soles. This thickness is predetermined embryologically and not primarily by pressure and trauma, though these factors can increase thickness. When transplanted, palmar or plantar skin continues to be "palmar" or "plantar" skin morphologically, no matter where it is placed.

The epidermis is ectodermal in origin. It consists entirely of cells (anywhere from ten layers of cells to several dozen). It contains no blood vessels or lymph channels and depends upon tissue fluid for its sustenance. It is the depository of the terminal ramifications of sensory nerve fibers and is anchored to the dermis by the papillae of the dermis with which it is functionally interdependent.

The epidermis contains two distinct cell types:

1. Keratinocytes which produce the fibrous protein keratin, possess A and B blood group antigens and share in some immune reactions.
2. Melanocytes, the melanin-forming cells.

The keratinocytes are most numerous and comprise 95 percent of the epidermis; the melanocytes make up the other 5 percent.

On microscopic examination, the epidermis is separated into five layers—basal, prickle, granular, stratum lucidum (visible only on the palms and soles) and horny—representing distinct functional stages in the keratinization process.

The basal layer is innermost and consists of a single row of columnar cells. Scattered among the cylindrical cells, there is also an interconnecting network of dendritic cells (melanocytes) that branch among and carry melanin pigment to the adjoining epidermal cells. Frequently, melanin granules form a supranuclear cap in the basal cells.

The basal layer is the progenitor of all the other cells in the epidermis. The main source of regenerative activity is from the basal layer; mitotic activity is greatest at night and is accelerated as a response to removal of the stratum corneum, injury and repair. The increase in cell population from normal mitotic activity produces a gradual outward displacement of all the cells toward the surface.

The prickle cell layer (stratum spinosum, malpighian layer) composes most of the epidermis and is made up of cells which are polygonal and form a mosaic. The cells are separated by spaces that are traversed by intercellular bridges or prickles. The spaces are perhaps functionally analogous to lymphatic vessels and play an important part in the nutrition and metabolic exchanges of the cells. Electron microscopy has demonstrated that the prickles are "attachment plaques" of the cell membranes of opposing cells; tonofibrils extend from the cytoplasm out to the plaques. The entire complex has been termed the desmosome.

The granular layer (stratum granulosum) consists of diamond-shaped cells filled with basophilic granules. The thickness of the stratum granulosum varies from one to three layers. It is most prominent where the degree of keratinization is least active. The cells are less hydrated, their nuclei are disorganized, and the intercellular bridges have all but disappeared.

The stratum lucidum is a narrow band of flattened cells which lack nuclei and is situated immediately beneath the horny layer. It is most prominent and visible on the palms and soles.

The horny layer (stratum corneum) is the outermost or surface layer of the epidermis. It is composed of compressed, parallel, homogenized, nonnucleated cells—dead epithelial cells that have become horny or keratinized. The lower part of the horny layer is compact and coherent (stratum compactum), but in its upper part the horny cells lose their coherence (stratum disjunctum).

Keratinization. The term keratinization denotes the morphologic and biochemical changes associated with the outward progress of cells from the basal layer to the horny layer. It has been estimated that it takes approximately 28 days for a cell to mature, that is to progress from basal layer to final shedding.

Keratinization is the synthesis of fibrous proteins made up of amino acids embedded in an amorphous ground substance. The sequence of amino acids along the polypeptide chains is probably significant in determining the type of keratin. Keratinization is not synonymous with horny layer formation. The horny layer contains about 50 percent of other materials, by-products of keratinization, along with keratin.

DERMIS

The dermis or corium, the connective-tissue layer, along with its blood vessels and nerves, supports and is intimately associated with the overlying epidermis and separates it from the subcutaneous fat.

The dermis makes up the bulk of the skin. It is divided into two sections: (1) stratum papillare, the most superficial portion which projects as finger-like extensions (called papillae or papillary bodies) into the epidermis, and (2) stratum reticulare, the lower portion. The main constituents of the dermis are the collagenous, elastic, and reticular fibers. Collagen makes up about 95 percent of the dermis. Elastic fibers are found entwined among the collagen bundles. Reticular fibers, probably immature collagen, present as a basket weave of fine elements. Occupying the spaces between fibers is the ground substance or matrix. Cellular elements consist of fibrocytes, histiocytes and mastocytes.

Collagen is a tough, resistant fibrous protein. Its amino acid composition shows a high content of glycine and lesser amounts of proline and hydroxyproline. Elastic fibers are composed of elastin, a protein similar to collagen but having important differences. The ground substance is a viscous material whose main constituents are the mucopolysaccharides, hyaluronic acid and chondroitin sulfate.

The dermis also contains a superficial (subpapillary) and a deep (reticular) vascular network, lymphatic capillaries and vessels which accompany the veins, autonomic and peripheral nerves.

HYPODERMIS

The subcutis (fatty layer) is the deepest skin layer and is characterized by closely packed lipocytes. This fatty layer varies in thickness and composition and shows a selective distribution throughout the body. By simple syringe biopsy technique, the composition of fat can be studied by gas-liquid chromatography for analysis of the adipose triglycerides.

SKIN APPENDAGES

Among the appendages, the sweat glands and nails are pertinent to the lower extremities. The ubiquitous eccrine sweat glands are coiled tubular glands situated at the dermal-subdermal junction with their ducts straightening out, piercing the dermis, and finally spiraling through the epidermis to the surface. Pertinent data relating to the eccrine glands are reviewed in the section under sweat disorders.

The nail organ is formed from an invagination of epidermis located on the dorsum of the distal phalanx of each digit. The invagination is first noted in the fetus at nine weeks and development of the nail plate is completed by the twentieth week. The nail is formed by the matrix located at the floor of the posterior nail fold. It grows forward instead of upward because of pressure from the posterior nail fold. Nails grow continuously throughout life at a rate of approximately 0.1 mm. per day, one-third the growth rate of hair. Toenails grow at one-third to one-half the rate of fingernails. There is also some variation in the precise growth rate of the nails of the various individual digits.

The formation of nail by the matrix is an active metabolic process and is therefore susceptible to local and systemic disorders. The nail plate is a dead structure and defects of the plate represent the "scars" of previous damage to the matrix occurring when that particular portion of nail was being formed.

The nail normally appears pink because of the reflection of light from the underlying capillary bed throughout the translucent nail. Normally the epithelium of the nail bed does not keratinize. If as a result of a pathologic process, the nail bed produces keratin, the nail appears white rather than pink.

The nail changes seen in various diseases of the feet will be described as each clinical disorder is discussed.

HISTOPATHOLOGIC FACTORS

Epidermis

Pathologic processes primarily involving the epidermis may be

1. Congenital: (a) generalized as ichthyosis
   (b) localized as keratoderma palmaris et plantaris
2. Acquired: (a) limited as a callus
   (b) diffuse as pityriasis rubra pilaris

Pathologic changes in the epidermis depend upon the involved cellular tissue: keratinocyte; melanocyte.

Keratinocyte

1. Alterations in function
   a. Hyperkeratosis: increased keratinocyte activity as seen in the corn or callus in which the hyperkeratosis is due to stimulation of the epidermis by intermittent pressure.
   b. Parakeratosis: accelerated keratinocyte activity, usually seen in association with inflammatory diseases of the skin. The resulting cells are not completely mature and therefore retain their nuclei.
   c. Dyskeratosis: imperfect keratinocyte activity or abnormal cornification as the benign disorder Darier's disease, or as a malignant change in Paget's disease of the nipple, Bowen's disease and squamous cell carcinoma.
2. Alterations from injury: the malpighian layer is the principal site and is characterized by the blistering diseases.
3. Alterations in growth
   a. Verrucae and seborrheic keratoses are simple examples of benign overgrowth of the keratinocyte.

b. Basal and squamous cell epitheliomas are the common malignancies involving the keratinocyte.

Melanocyte

1. Alterations in function
    a. Hyperfunction: postinflammatory hyperpigmentation, tanning, freckles, chloasma.
    b. Loss of pigment: vitiligo, leukoderma.

Corium

Pathologic changes in the corium are innumerable; in general, they may be described according to cellular connective tissue, and matrix.

Cellular Changes. Simple inflammations: acute or chronic; granulomas; neoplasias.

1. Acute inflammations: characterized by a perivascular infiltration usually about the pilosebaceous apparatus and sweat glands. The infiltrate is usually composed of polymorphonuclear leukocytes. Lymphocytes predominate in subacute and chronic inflammations; in deeper chronic inflammations, plasma cells are increased.
2. Granulomas: the cellular infiltrations characteristic of a limited number of slowly progressive, persistent diseases. Granulomas consist of plasma cells, epithelioid cells and multinucleated giant cells.
    a. Nonspecific granulomas: from chronic mechanical or chemical irritation (i.e., poor-fitting shoes, purulent exudates).
    b. Foreign body granulomas.
    c. Infectious granulomas: syphilis, leprosy, tuberculosis, sarcoidosis and deep mycoses.

The infectious granulomas have certain distinctive histologic features: for example, plasma cells in syphilis, lepra cells in leprosy, tubercles in tuberculosis, abscesses and sinuses in addition to plasma cells in mycotic granulomas.

3. Neoplasms (tumor cells): those primary in the corium are characterized by cellular infiltrations that conform to the cells of origin of their lineage. They may be benign or malignant: the fibroma is a benign alteration; the fibrosarcoma and reticulum cell sarcoma are malignant changes in the connective tissue cells. Carcinomas resemble those of either the basal cell or prickle cell layer of the epidermis, or may be mixed. About the invading edge of most malignant tumors, there is a tissue reaction consisting of plasma cells and leucocytes.

    In melanomas, the tumor cells contain large, irregularly densely stained nuclei and nucleoli, the greatest activity being at the dermoepidermal junction.

Alterations in the Connective Tissue

1. Elastic fibers — may be degenerated, scarce or absent (scars). In atrophic skin, the elastic fibers show marked changes, and fatty or calcareous deposits may occur.
2. Collagenous fibers — may be subject to a variety of chemical degenerative changes which give rise to altered staining reactions.

Changes in the Matrix. They relate to chemical alterations in hyaluronic acid and chondroitin sulfate.

Hypodermis

Pathologic Changes in the Fatty Layer. These changes are divided into:

1. Noninflammatory disorders such as low-protein edema (cardiac, renal), high-protein edema (lymphedema, elephantiasis) and cold injury (immersion foot).
2. Inflammatory disorders such as traumatic (mechanical, physical or chemical), infective (tuberculosis, syphilis, leprosy), pancreatic disease and uncertain etiology such as erythema nodosum, nodular vasculitis or Weber-Christian disease.

Common Histopathologic Terms. Acanthosis — an increase in the thickness of the prickle cell or malpighian layer.

Hyperkeratosis — an increase in the thickness of the stratum corneum or horny layer.

Liquefaction degeneration of basal cells — destruction of the basal cells by vacuolization as seen in lupus erythematosus, dermatomyositis and lichen sclerosus et atrophicus.

Parakeratosis — incomplete keratinization due to the rapid migration of the prickle cells from the basal layer to the horny layer. Because of this immaturity of the cell, the nuclei are retained in the stratum corneum.

Spongiosis — edema between the individual prickle cells causing widening of the space between them (intercellular edema). This change is seen most often in inflammatory disorders, especially eczematous dermatitides.

STRUCTURE AND FUNCTION OF THE SKIN

As man descended, he evolved two critical cutaneous adaptations: loss of most of his body hair and the development of eccrine sweat glands which serve a thermoregulatory function. These evolutionary changes resulted in increased freedom of movement, but at the expense of protection. For man to survive in his environment, it was essential that he evolve adaptations of his cutaneous integument to provide an effective barrier against the continuous onslaught of radiation, chemicals and microorganisms to which he is subjected and to prevent loss of water to the external environment. The human skin has successfully developed this bidirectional barrier function, thus, preventing the egress of water and the ingress of noxious environmental agents.

Protection against mechanical trauma is provided by a two-phase integumentary system — tough yet resilient fibers imbedded in a pliable matrix — which is present throughout all layers of the skin. The stratum corneum provides a protective external barrier of great toughness over the entire body surface. The principal function of the epidermis is the replacement of the stratum corneum cells that are being continuously worn away or shed. In protecting against chemical agents, the horny layer acts as a physical barrier. Through the darkening of pigment precursors, the subsequent increased production and migration of melanin and the later thickening of the horny layer, the skin achieves some measure of protection against ultraviolet radiation.

The dermis is composed of collagen and elastin fibers within a ground substance matrix. It functions as a support for the epidermis and binds the epidermis so that it conforms to the underlying tissues.

Diffusely distributed throughout the dermis and subcutaneous fat tissue is an abundant network of blood vessels providing the skin with a blood supply far in excess of its metabolic needs. The function of this rich vasculature is temperature regulation. Upon exposure to cold, the cutaneous blood flow is decreased by the vasoconstrictor effects of stimulation of sympathetic nerve endings and heat is thereby retained. Conversely, an inhibition of the sympathetic nerve discharges upon exposure to heat leads to cutaneous vasodilatation and increased heat loss. If this mechanism fails to maintain a normal body temperature, the eccrine sweat glands increase their activity and body heat is dissipated through the evaporation of water from the skin surface. (For further information concerning the cutaneous vascular system, refer to Hunting Reaction, page 73.)

The subcutaneous fat layer below the dermis provides a measure of insulation, protecting the body from excess external heat and decreasing heat loss when exposed to the cold.

The mechanisms by which the skin protects against bacteria are still somewhat controversial but desiccation appears to be the main defense against *E. coli* and *Pseudomonas.* In the case of streptococci, the antibacterial action of fatty acids, particularly oleic seems most effective. An additional, and possibly very important, factor in protection of the skin against pathogenic microorganisms, is the phenomenon of bacterial interference; for example, the presence of one strain of staphylococci at a cutaneous site prevents colonization of that location by another strain.

REGIONAL VARIATIONS IN ANATOMY AND FUNCTION

It is clear to even the most casual observer that there are marked differences in the skin of the palms and soles as compared to glabrous skin elsewhere on the body.

The horny layer of the palms and soles is markedly thickened, measuring up to 1.0 mm., in contrast to the stratum corneum elsewhere which usually is about 10 microns in thickness. In the palms and soles the deeper portion of the stratum corneum, the stratum lucidum, is present as a distinct layer which is not noted in skin from other sites. This markedly thickened horny layer occasionally lends a yellowish appearance to lesions leading to a possible mistaken clinical diagnosis of xanthomata. The thick stratum corneum also necessitates that biopsies of the palms or soles be much deeper than those taken from skin elsewhere.

Apocrine glands, sebaceous glands and hair are absent from the palms and soles while eccrine glands are numerous. The ability of the skin of these areas to maintain a "grip" and avoid slippage is related to the absence of oil or hair and is due to the presence of moisture from the sweat glands.

The skin of the palms and soles, though distinctly different from that of other portions of the body, is quite similar. However, as pointed out by Marples,[1] our bipedal style of locomotion produces totally different environmental conditions in the two areas. The hands are freely exposed, are in wide ranging motion and the digits are relatively separated and mobile. By contrast, the feet are encased in rather impervious shoes, their movement is relatively restricted, large areas of the skin are compressed by the body weight and the toes are fairly immobile. The skin temperature of the feet is lower than that of any other body area. The thick stratum corneum of the feet can absorb large quantities of water and evaporation is decreased by the low skin temperature and the impervious coverings. These factors lead to maceration and an alkaline pH which in turn favor the establishment of dermatophytes. Fungi are rarely isolated from the feet of people who habitually go barefoot whereas they are recovered with such regularity from the feet of people who wear shoes that they might almost be considered as part of the normal flora of the toe webs.

DERMATOGLYPHICS

Dermatoglyphics are furrows in the skin of the digital pads, palms and soles and can be permanently recorded on specially treated paper by various techniques of imprinting. Fingerprinting has been known and utilized as a method of identification for years; however, more recently this procedure has become useful in clinical medicine and genetics. The differentiation of the skin ridges occurs in the developing fetus between the thirteenth and nineteenth weeks, with the hand developing somewhat earlier than the foot.

Dermatoglyphic patterns of the fingers and palms have been studied extensively in many disease states. The mechanism of their production is still not completely clear. Abnormalities have been described in such congenital disorders resulting from chromosomal defects as mongolism, Trisomy D, Trisomy E, cri-du-chat, XXYY, XYY, and Klinefelter's syndrome and in such miscellaneous disorders as in-utero infection with rubella, psoriasis, von Recklinghausen's disease, pseudohypoparathyroidism, Wilson's disease and schizophrenia.

In recent years, since the discovery of abnormal patterns of the ball area of the sole in cases of chromosomal anomalies, greater attention has been directed toward the dermatoglyphic patterns occurring on the sole. Abnormalities have been reported in such conditions as anonychia, nail-patella syndrome, zygodactyly, syndactyly, brachydactyly, polydactyly, Down's syndrome (mongolism), Trisomy 13, 14 or 15, 17 or 18, Turner's syndrome and Klinefelter's syndrome. A clinical diagnosis however should not be made on dermatoglyphic features alone. (For detailed discussion of the normal and abnormal dermatoglyphic patterns of the sole, the reader is referred to Holt[2] and Cummins and Midlo.[3])

PLANTAR SKIN AS A RESEARCH TOOL

The skin of the foot, particularly the callus, can be utilized to study many aspects of cutaneous physiology, biochemistry and microbiology including keratinization, blister formation and percutaneous absorption.

Keratinization

A major function of the epidermis is the production of keratin. Keratin is often classed as either soft, as in human skin, or hard, as in hair, horns, and so on. Keratins are fibrous proteins resistant to enzymatic digestion and to hydrolysis by acids and alkalis. They are crystalline structures whose atoms are arranged in a regular repetitive pattern resulting in an x-ray diffraction pattern of an alpha type; when the normally folded keratin polypeptide chains are stretched, the x-ray pattern is of a beta configuration. Keratin has a high cystine content and the level of cystine parallels the degree of hardness of the keratin. Since the production of keratin is the paramount function of the epidermis and the maturation of the epidermal cells is paralleled by the appearance of keratin within the cells, further study of keratin will provide better understanding of the structure and function of the skin.

Callus

Numerous studies of cutaneous physiology and biochemistry have been carried out utilizing readily available callus. It has been legitimately questioned how applicable such results are to normal glabrous skin; nevertheless, studies using callus have yielded much worthwhile information. A very important basic finding was that dry callus remains hard and brittle in the presence of petrolatum or other oils but becomes soft and pliable if allowed to absorb some water. (For further information consult the classic studies of I.H. Blank.[4,5])

Friction Blisters

Friction blisters are distinctive forms of reactions confined to the human species. These lesions occur with frequency and constitute one of man's commonest reactions to trauma, especially of the lower extremities. Studies have shown that extremes of dryness and wetness tend to decrease friction, whereas intermediate degrees of moisture at the rubbing surface tend to increase skin friction. Friction blisters do not usually occur clinically on thin skin because it lacks the thick and resistant stratum corneum for the blister roof. They also do not usually occur on loose skin because it lacks the tight adherence of the skin to underlying structures necessary for shearing effects to be produced in the epidermis. An intact arterial circulation and an adequate hemodynamic pressure are required for free fluid to accumulate in the area damaged by the shearing forces. Recent studies by Sulzberger and his colleagues[6,7] have yielded significant information and pointed out new areas for further research activities.

Percutaneous Absorption

A vital function of the skin is to act as a barrier — to prevent the absorption inward of noxious substances and to retard the outward passage of water. However, the effectiveness of this barrier function varies depending upon the material presented to the skin and upon other environmental factors present at the time. Thus, the presence of moisture increases absorption, surfactants increase absorption; the absorption of acidic and basic drugs will be greatly influenced by the pH of the vehicle. Thickness of the skin and its temperature also affect the rate of absorption.

There is still much debate concerning the routes of absorption through the skin. Essentially there are two routes, the transepidermal and the transappendageal (through the hair follicles, sweat glands and sebaceous glands). Many observers now feel that early transient percutaneous absorption is through the hair follicles and ducts and steady state diffusion is primarily through the intact stratum corneum.

Numerous investigators, including Stoughton[8] and Scheuplein,[9] have contributed to our present knowledge of percutaneous absorption. Despite these excellent studies, however, much remains to be elucidated about the barrier function of the skin. Such information has much practical importance, for intelligent formulation of dermatological preparations depends upon a thorough understanding of percutaneous absorption.

References

1. Marples, M.J.: The Ecology of the Human Skin. p. 182. Springfield, (Ill.), Charles C Thomas, 1965.
2. Holt, S.B.: The Genetics of Dermal Ridges. Springfield, (Ill.), Charles C Thomas, 1968.
3. Cummins, H., and Midlo, C.: Fingerprints, Palms and Soles. An Introduction to Dermatoglyphics. New York, Dover Publications, Inc. 1961.
4. Blank, I.H.: Factors which influence the water content of the stratum corneum. J. Invest. Derm., *18*:433, 1952.
5. Blank, I.H.: Further observations on factors which influence the water content of the stratum corneum. J. Invest. Derm., *21*:259, 1953.
6. Sulzberger, M.B., Cortese, T.A., Fishman, L., and Wiley, H.S.: Studies on blisters produced by friction I. Results of linear rubbing and twisting technics. J. Invest. Derm., *47*:456, 1966.
7. Cortese, T.A., Sams, W.M., and Sulzberger, M.B.: Studies on blisters produced by friction II. The blister fluid. J. Invest. Derm., *50*:47, 1968.
8. Stoughton, R.B.: Some *in vivo* and *in vitro* methods for measuring percutaneous absorption. *In* Rook, A., and Champion, R.H. (eds.): Progress in the Biological Sciences in Relation to Dermatology-2. pp. 263-274. London, Cambridge University Press, 1964.
9. Scheuplein, R.J.: Mechanism of percutaneous absorption II. Transient diffusion and the relative importance of various routes of skin penetration. J. Invest. Derm., *48*:79, 1967.

PRINCIPLES OF DIAGNOSIS

The basic mechanisms of dermatologic disease will be better understood when we learn more about genetics, molecular biology, biochemistry and physiology. Until this information is forthcoming, we shall have to concern ourselves with morphology and classification.

A practical approach to establishing an etiologic diagnosis utilizes the following:

1. Clinical findings
2. Histopathologic and histochemical studies
3. Laboratory studies
4. Special dermatological procedures and skin tests

CLINICAL FINDINGS (History, Lesions, Topography)

History

A well-planned history is often essential for an etiologic diagnosis. One starts with the chief complaint, the date and site of onset, possible precipitating factors, the presence or absence of subjective symptoms, course, exacerbations and recurrences. With experience, the history can be effectively directed. At times, these data may be sufficient to make a diagnosis. More often, an extensive thorough questioning will be necessary and may have to be reexplored at subsequent interviews. The following represent some aspects of the historical data.

Family History. The traditional history of the general health, or causes of death of parents and siblings, is of obvious importance. There is probably some genetic factor in almost all disease processes, but the extent of this component varies. The spectrum embraces rare disorders such as ichthyosis, Mal de Meleda, epidermolysis bullosa, thalassemia, sickle cell anemia, porokeratosis of Mibelli, certain common skin diseases such as atopic dermatitis and psoriasis, and systemic diseases such as diabetes. Certain diseases such as scabies, furunculosis and tuberculosis may show a high familial incidence without being hereditary.

Personal History. A history of systemic disease, recent and current illnesses and past dermatological illness probably provide helpful diagnostic clues. Certain skin diseases of the lower extremities are prone to affect particular age groups; for example, atopic dermatitis and papular urticaria in childhood and adolescence, pigmented purpuric eruptions, xerosis and skin cancer in older people. Sex is an important determinant; for example, tinea pedis and Kaposi's sarcoma occur dominantly in males. Erythema induratum and lupus erythematosus mainly affect females.

Geographic Origin and Travel. Certain diseases are endemic in different areas of the world; for example, leprosy in the Philippines, China, India, Cuba, Espanol and South America; leishmaniasis in Israel, Iran and other Near East countries, kwashiorkor in Africa and South America, miliaria in the tropics, chigger bites in southern United States, poison ivy dermatitis in the eastern half of the United States. Therefore, the present and past places of residence, as well as time spent in different areas on holidays and on long travel trips may be significant. "Tropical" diseases are appearing with increasing frequency among travelers who live in temperate zones.

Season of Year. Seasons may strikingly influence skin disease. Atopic dermatitis has spring and fall flares. Contact dermatitis due to plants largely occurs in spring and summer. Typical summer problems include insect bites, photosensitivity, miliaria; ragweed dermatitis occurs in the early autumn; winter brings chapping, xerosis and pruritus.

Occupation and Avocation. In this list are the physical, biological and chemical agents responsible for occupational dermatoses, the irritant and sensitizing chemical compounds contacted in our leisure activities, the reactions due to cosmetics and wearing apparel, and environmental exposures such as pesticides and cleansers. The most detailed interrogation may be necessary to establish a causal relationship.

Previous Medications. One must always be alert to the fact that the presenting skin lesions may be due to drugs. Almost any drug can cause an adverse reaction in certain persons. These drugs include self-medications, patent medicines and those prescribed to be taken orally, by inhalation and by injection. One can include in this category the host of flavorings and preservatives in various foods and the chemicals in soft drinks and foods. Adverse reactions from drugs such as antibiotics, analgesics, soporifics, tranquilizers, diuretics and other common medicaments are common. Less frequently recognized are the many drugs capable of triggering photosensitivity reactions; for example thiazides in diuretics, certain antibiotics (Declomycin, tetracycline), sulfonamides, tranquilizers (Thorazine), antiseptics (bithionol), antihistaminics (Phenergan), oral hypoglycemic agents (Diabinese, Orinase) and griseofulvin. Of great importance is information relating to topical forms of treatment the patient had already used for his skin problem including such measures as x-ray and ultraviolet light therapy, and medicaments used in the form of ointments, creams, lotions or sprays. Common offenders are antibiotics, antihistaminics, fungicides and local anesthetics. Reactions may be produced not only by the active chemical constituents in these medications but also by the vehicles and preservatives.

Psychological Factors. Every skin disorder may have an associated emotional component. What is germane is to determine which feature is primary and to assess the exact role that the psychological factors play in the presenting symptoms. Emotions probably have been overemphasized in the causation of disorders which still remain unexplained. Anxiety is usually a consequence not a cause of the skin disease.

Lesions

Careful inspection of the skin and characterization of the lesions provide the basis for developing the diagnosis. "Lesions are the alphabet without which nobody can read the language of the skin" (Darier). Meaningful concepts can be crystallized from these observations; at times this alone is adequate for diagnosis. Proper examination of the skin always requires good lighting, preferably daylight. Adequate exposure of the entire skin and systematic examination is frequently necessary. The oral mucous membrane should be examined routinely.

There are three types of lesions: primary, secondary and elementary. Primary lesions, which reflect the direct expression of the disease process, are macule, petechia, papule, nodule, wheal, vesicle and bulla, pustule, tumor. Secondary lesions are scales, crusts, excoriations, fissures, erosions, ulcers, scars and atrophy. However the differentiation is not always clear. The so-called elementary lesions, comedo, milium, burrow, lichenification and telangiectasis, are instances of unique skin reactions.

The fact that one can diagnose a skin lesion is important; however, one must try to understand the mechanism responsible for its formation. *Why* did the lesion become manifest? Is there an external cause—a chemical, an insect, a fungus, a bacterium? Is the skin lesion part of a systemic disorder as in dermatomyositis and lupus erythematosus? Is the skin reacting to an underlying abnormality; for example, bullae with porphyria, aphthae and pyoderma gangrenosum with ulcerative colitis? Is the lesion a presenting symptom of a strictly dermatologic entity as in psoriasis and lichen planus?

What are the possible biochemical changes or physiological alterations responsible for the structural change which manifests as the presenting lesion? *Why* in the alteration of function did such a structural change take place? Why was a macule the resultant lesion and not a vesicle or papule? Why was a crust formed and not a scale? *How* was such a lesion formed? Was something done on the exposed surface or was something wrong internally? Is this lesion congenital or was it acquired? Is it of a temporary nature or will it be permanent?

Some of these aspects can be elucidated almost at a glance, others require extensive additional studies. In essence, we see the effect, so we must search for the cause.

Macule. A circumscribed alteration in the color of the skin, not visibly raised, or depressed, or presenting any change in the consistency of the skin. Macules may be due to changes in blood vessels; for example, hyperemic or inflammatory macules which are transient dilatations of blood vessels, and nevi such as nevus flammeus and nevus anemicus are the permanent enlargement or absence of blood vessels respectively. Macules may also be due to changes in pigment (melanin), either to deficiency such as in vitiligo; or to an increase such as the café au lait mark, freckle or fixed drug eruption; or to infection such as tinea versicolor; or to depositions in the skin produced internally by bile pigments, blood pigments and iron; or externally such as from gunpowder or maculae cerulae; or to coloration produced by internal factors such as argyria and atabrine dermatitis and exogenous causes such as from silver nitrate.

Papule. A small elevation above the skin level. A papule has a solid center and can be felt, although on the palms and soles it is often flattened by pressure. It varies in size from a millimeter to a centimeter and its shape depends upon the level of the underlying infiltrate. Papules may be produced by an increase in cells in the horny layer—warts; by edema in the epidermis—eczema; by edema, inflammatory changes or cellular infiltrates in the dermis—lichen planus, tuberculids and papular syphilids.

Nodule. A solid lesion larger than a papule and consisting of inflammatory cellular infiltrates (e.g., erythema nodosum and erythema induratum), neoplasms (e.g., epitheliomata or tissue hypertrophies). Nodular lesions frequently show a destructive character and break down with suppuration (e.g., gummas, erythema induratum and Weber-Christian disease).

Wheal (Hive). An evanescent plateau-like elevation produced by edema in the upper corium and the extravasation of blood plasma through the vessel walls. Whealing or urtication may be produced either by external causes—reactions to insect bites or allergic responses to scratch and intracutaneous tests—or by internal factors—drug and food allergy. Wheals may be the same color as normal skin, redder if the superficial blood vessels are dilated and paler if the blood vessels are compressed by the extravasated fluid.

Vesicle. A circumscribed elevation of the skin containing fluid, a blister. Microscopically vesicles vary in their pathogenesis and can be distinguished as subcorneal, intraepidermal and subepidermal. Impetigo presents as subcorneal separation; primary cell damage (intracellular) with ballooning cell forms is often due to virus invasion. Intercellular edema (spongiosis) is typical of contact dermatitis. Completely separated epidermal cells with loss of intercellular bridges is termed acantholysis of which the classical example is pemphigus. Subepidermal vesicles result from the separation between the epidermis and corium (e.g., dermatitis herpetiformis, bullous pemphigoid, erythema multiforme and epidermolysis bullosa). Vesicles are spherical and are characterized by their roofs, contents and bases. They are usually tense and have a taut surface. If imbedded in thick skin, as in that of the palms and soles, they may be neither raised nor palpable.

Bulla. A large vesicle. Bullae are produced by extrinsic factors such as chemical (cantharides, adhesive), thermic (burns, frostbite), mechanical (friction) or by internal factors as in erythema multiforme, pemphigus, pemphigoid and porphyria.

Pustule. A circumscribed liquid accumulation containing free pus. Sometimes pustules start as vesicles such as staphylococcic infection (vesiculo-pustules). Primary pustules are seen with such inflammations as folliculitis, periporitis, ecthyma, pustular psoriasis, pustular bacterids, acrodermatitis continua and subcorneal pustulosis.

Tumors. A new growth of varying size composed of skin and subcutaneous tissue. Tumors may be benign (lipomas and fibromas) or malignant (basal and prickle cell epitheliomas, sarcomas, lymphomas).

Scales. The exfoliation of accumulated debris of dead stratum corneum and result from imperfect cornification. Scales are characterized by their color (e.g., the silvery or mica-like scales of psoriasis, loose or dry of exfoliative dermatitis and ichthyosis, greasy of seborrheic dermatitis and Darier's disease, branny of *T. rubrum* infections and pityriasis rubra pilaris, adherent of discoid lupus erythematosus and actinic keratoses).

Crusts. Result from the drying of fluid, pus, serum, and blood in combination with scales, dirt and bacteria on or in skin. Crusts may be thick, thin, bloody or necrotic.

Excoriation. The loss of superficial substance of the skin as the result of scratching. Exposure of the corium and bleeding result from the mechanical removal of the epidermis.

Fissure. Lines or grooves due to the loss of continuity of the skin without any loss of substance. Normal fissures are preformed on the palms and soles; acquired fissures represent the loss of elasticity sequential usually to an inflammatory infiltrate.

Erosions. A denuded area due to the loss of all or part of the epidermis. Erosions are often the result of trauma to a primary lesion such as a vesicle or maceration secondary to ringworm of the toes. An erosion sequential to a bulla frequently presents a circular outline with a collarette of scales. Some postbullous erosions form vegetations instead of healing smoothly.

Ulcers. Produced by a destruction of skin with resultant scar formation. Ulcers are described by their size, depth, number and by such features as induration and presence of underlying lesions. (See causes of ulcers on the lower extremities, in Chap. 8.)

Scars. Alterations of skin following destruction of the epidermis and cutis. Some scars become hypertrophic, of which keloids are a prominent example. They tend to occur in Negroes in certain areas of the body especially the sternum. Hypertrophic scars are frequently provoked by burns. Irregular scars develop in syphilis and acne conglobata. New scars are pinkish in color; old ones white and shiny.

Atrophy. Implies loss of tissue; either all or some of the tissues of the skin. Fragmentation and degeneration of the elastic tissue is a common pathological finding. It is clinically manifested by a diminution of the actual thickness of the skin. Atrophic skin is more supple and thinner than normal skin, shows fine wrinkling, puckers like tissue paper, and has a parchment feel. Its color is pinkish to pearly white. Atrophy of the skin may be congenital (e.g., congenital ectodermal defect and pseudoxanthoma elasticum). The acquired forms of atrophy may follow damage to the skin as from x-ray dermatitis or from senile atrophy where the degenerative changes are caused by sunlight. Striae (linear atrophy) may follow cachexia and obesity or may be induced by the administration of ACTH, at sites of application of topical corticosteroids or in pituitary diseases. Post-traumatic or post-ulcerative types of atrophy appear as the final stages of interstitial pathologic processes. Many atrophic lesions are of unknown etiology (e.g., the various macular atrophies, the diffuse picture of acrodermatitis chronica atrophicans, the poikilodermas, kraurosis vulvae, balanitis xerotica obliterans and lichen sclerosus et atrophicus).

Lichenification. Infiltration of the skin horizontally rather than in depth producing a thickened skin with accentuated skin markings. The surface relief presents a coarsened appearance similar to that of shagreen. The color of lichenified skin may be red, more frequently pale and somewhat grayish. After a time, hyperpigmentation develops and may extend to the surrounding skin.

Telangiectasis. Visibly dilated, superficial blood vessels seen in connection with certain heritable diseases such as familial telangiectasis, associated with liver diseases and pregnancy and as a sequel to x-ray treatment.

Skin lesions have certain attributes which are helpful in making a diagnosis.

Color Changes

The color of normal skin takes its origin from the pigments in various layers and from the state and amount of blood in the superficial vascular plexuses.

A. **Pigments.** *Natural pigments* include melanin, carotene, bile and occasionally pigments in apocrine sweat. Localized increase of melanin occurs in freckles, chloasma, certain nevi, café au lait spots, Peutz-Jeghers syndrome and in post-inflammatory reactions, viz, pyodermas, psoriasis, lichen planus and syphilis. Decrease in melanin occurs in nevi depigmentosa, vitiligo and after inflammation. Carotenemia represents an increase in carotene; jaundice reflects an increase in bile pigments.

Foreign pigments—tattoos are the best examples. The color tells the pigment—green due to chromates, red due to cinnabar and carmine, gray-black hues from gunpowder or pictures peculiar to certain occupations such as that of miners and stonemasons.

Drugs taken internally can produce color changes; for example, the slate-gray color of argyria due to silver, the yellow color of atabrine, the dusky gray-purple color of thorazine and Declomycin following sun exposure, the blue-gray line of the gums from bismuth.

Drugs applied externally may cause color changes; for example, tar, chrysarobin, anthralin.

Foreign Cells. Examples of characteristic color changes are the lemon yellow scutulum of favus, blackening of the horny layer due to dirt implanted in cracks and calluses on hands and feet.

Blood. Depositions of hemosiderin give rise to petechia, purpura, and ecchymosis.

Cells and cellular products. Cellular products in representative lesions of certain diseases show characteristic color tones: yellow-orange (xanthomatosis and necrobiosis lipoidica diabeticorum), ham (secondary syphilis), violaceus (lichen planus), silvery shades (psoriasis), red-brown or red-blue (lupus pernio color) (sarcoid and tuberculoid lesions), black (black hairy tongue).

B. **Blood Color.**

Color changes follow hyperemia or vasomotor changes; for example, erythema, cutis marmorata. Permanent increase or enlargement of blood vessels; for example, telangiectasis, angiomata, spider nevi, nevus flammeus, livedo reticularis.

Spatial Relationships of Lesions

Lesions present in different configurations. They may be solitary, discrete, grouped or herpetic, aggregate or confluent. Lesions are described as localized or circumscribed, diffuse, generalized and universal. A uniform eruption describes lesions of the same type. The term multiform, or polymorphous, is used for different types of lesions in the same eruption.

Descriptive Terms Relating to Lesions

Knowledgeable use of these terms provides a picture of what the lesion actually looks like.

Size

This should be expressed in millimeters and centimeters.

Shape and Configuration

They may appear round, oval, polygonal, square or irregular, linear, acuminate, filiform, spinulose, umbilicated, imbricated, rupial, condylomatous, vegetative, papillomatous, iris, serpiginous, circumscribed, discoid, circinate, annular, retiform, punctate, nummular, plaque.

Contents

The contents may be sweat, sebum, lymph, blood, horny material, foreign material.

Topography

In this text we have restricted ourselves to those diseases localized on the lower extremities. The known causes and speculations of this selective distribution have been considered in the first part of this chapter.

HISTOPATHOLOGICAL AND HISTOCHEMICAL STUDIES

Histologic examination of the lesion is often necessary for diagnosis. Microscopic morphology may be diagnostically conclusive. The lesions are removed by a punch biopsy or scalpel excision, fixed, cut and stained. Hematoxylin and eosin are almost universally used for routine work but at times, special stains may be required.

Depending upon the history and clinical features, the clinician can request special studies which will utilize selective staining for histochemical alterations to identify special chemical substances (e.g., glycogen, amyloid and mucopolysaccharides).

Biopsies should be selective, that is, a representative lesion should be chosen. At times, multiple biopsies may be advisable. The ease with which skin biopsies can be performed enables the clinician to utilize them readily to assist in obtaining correct diagnosis. Unnecessary biopsies on the lower extremities should be avoided because of delayed healing in these areas, especially in patients over the age of forty with peripheral vascular or degenerative diseases.

LABORATORY STUDIES

Blood counts, urinalysis and serologic tests for syphilis have been standard laboratory tests. Routine studies of the sedimentation rate, blood sugar, blood urea nitrogen or serum uric acid may be indicated. Lesions in association with autoimmune diseases will require tests for rheumatoid factor, L. E. cells, electrophoretic patterns and fluorescent antibody studies. In connection with myositis, serum enzyme activity and electromyographic studies may be necessary. A battery of lipid studies are essential for the lipoproteinemias. Special blood studies are required for anemias and lymphoblastomas; sophisticated biochemical studies for genetic disorders. In some instances, x-ray examination of joint, bone, lung or gastrointestinal tract may be pertinent. In short, in any skin lesion which purports or reflects a systemic disease, use of the appropriate laboratory tests to give solid scientific support to the clinical judgment is imperative.

SPECIAL DERMATOLOGICAL PROCEDURES AND SKIN TESTS

Diagnostic clues:

Auspitz sign. The appearance of pinpoint bleeding when the scale of a lesion of psoriasis is forcibly removed.

Nikolsky sign. The upper layers of the epidermis easily detached by slight pressure or trauma, pointing to an absence of cohesion in the skin. The sign is elicited in pemphigus.

Koebner or isomorphic phenomenon. The production of lesions, by physical trauma, of the same form that is characteristic of the eruption. Commonly observed in psoriasis and lichen planus.

Touching, feeling and probing of lesions. To determine induration, thickening, atrophy, dryness, anesthesia and caseation.

Diascopy (glass pressure). To determine presence of intravascular blood and pigmentations and to detect the apple-jelly color in granulomatous lesions (e.g., lupus vulgaris). Lesions that consist of functioning blood vessels usually disappear under this procedure.

Cytodiagnosis.

1. Tzanck test for bullous diseases and for vesicular virus eruptions such as zoster, herpes simplex, varicella, molluscum contagiosum.
2. Suspected basal cell epitheliomas.

Examination of skin scrapings by direct microscopy. Tineas. See Chapter 2.

Cultures. Mycological, bacteriological, virological.

Use of ultraviolet light. To test for photosensitivity.

Wood's light. Erythrasma, tinea versicolor.

Exposure to cold and heat. To test for cold and heat hypersensitivity, Raynaud's phenomenon.

Skin testing.

1. Patch test.
2. Immediate: Wheal test (scratch and intradermal) for atopic dermatitis.
3. Delayed intradermal tests (tuberculin, trichophytin, antigens of the deep mycoses such as histoplasmin, coccidioidin).
4. Long-delayed intradermal tests (Kveim, Mitsuda).

Skin window technique. A small area of skin is gently abraded and a coverslip applied but is removed at intervals and replaced by another. The coverslips are stained and the cellular response can be evaluated.

Iontophoresis. A method of introducing into the skin substances which are ionized and carry an electric charge. Used as a research tool.

Immunofluorescent techniques have been of great aid in the diagnosis of certain cutaneous disorders. Specific staining patterns are observed in pemphigus vulgaris, bullous pemphigoid and lupus erythematosus.

With proper training, this data lends to computerization; correct feeding into the computer—presently, the brain, will piece the clues together to establish a diagnosis.

2

Microbiological Diseases

BASIC MICROBIOLOGY OF LOWER LEG SKIN*

Microbiological studies of the lower leg are best understood from the ecological standpoint. A variety of different microbial species exist on the surface of the skin under environments ranging from the dry calf to the wet toe webs. These species include potential pathogens, even in the absence of lesions, which are prevented from multiplying to high densities by other members of the microbial community. Disturbance of the ecological balance may occur spontaneously, or because of changes in the host affecting the microbial environment or as a result of therapy. The concept of a complex interacting flora changing as a result of outside influences, but retaining a strong homeostatic tendency, must replace the concept of one organism always causing one disease.[1]

Although the flora of the toe webs includes many species, many organisms in the general environment fail to colonize the skin. On the drier lower leg the flora is quite restricted due to the physical and chemical conditions on the surface and to the activities of the organisms already present. Different species differ in tolerance to dryness, pH changes, temperature and specific and nonspecific chemical inhibitors, such as fatty acids from the skin[2] and serum factors. The relative importance of these factors in controlling the composition and density of the normal flora varies from site to site, but the overwhelming importance of moisture in favoring increased density over most of the skin has been well demonstrated.[3,4]

The density and species variety of the toe webs appear to be greater than in the axilla where more than 10^6 bacteria per sq. cm. can be recovered.[5] On the calf, the quantity of organisms is similar to the forearm, about 10^3 organisms per sq. cm. The occurrence of *Corynebacterium minutissimum*, lipophilic and nonlipophilic diphtheroids, enterobacteria, *Pseudomonas*, *Mima-Herellea* and *Candida* species in the toe webs and axilla contrasts markedly with the dense coccal, *Corynebacterium acnes* flora of the head and the sparse coccal-lipophilic diphtheroid flora of the abdomen, leg and arm.

A high density of a complex flora in intertriginous areas produces a higher pH than elsewhere. Urea and other nitrogenous compounds are metabolized with the release of ammonia, while the low availability of carbohydrates prevents much acid production. This contrasts with Marchionini's thesis of a protective "acid mantle" preventing colonization of the skin.

*Contributed by Dr. Richard R. Marples, Department of Dermatology, University of Pennsylvania.

The low temperature of the lower extremity may also significantly alter the microbial flora. Some pathogens are unable to tolerate local temperatures of 37° C. Thus *Mycobacterium marinum* and dermatophytes can flourish in an area which rarely becomes hotter than 35° and is usually 4 or 5 degrees cooler while many recognized pathogens cannot multiply.[6] The very large number of non-lipophilic diphtheroids in the toe webs which are only rarely recovered from the much warmer axilla may also be due to the low temperature.

Topography and Nutrients

The relative importance of the substrate seems less in the lower extremities than elsewhere. The detailed anatomy of the skin surface is very similar to that of the arm. However, because of the custom of wearing shoes and the necessity for weight bearing, the local conditions of the skin are different, leading to retention of skin products, particularly water. The amount of fatty material from sebaceous glands arriving on the sole is less than on the palm. From this a greater incidence of streptococci might be expected, but is not seen. It has been suggested, though not proven, that low fatty acids on the foot may promote ringworm infection.[7] The lack of hairs in the toe webs and sole does not seem to diminish bacterial density, as would be expected if most bacteria inhabit the infundibular portion of hair follicles.[8]

Interspecific Interactions

Because a very dense normal flora is carried on the moist skin of the toe webs, interactions between microorganisms have been clearly demonstrated in this region. Combined occupation by dermatophytes, *Staphylococcus aureus* and *Candida albicans* intensifies itching and aggravates the inflammatory response.[9] Protection against colonization by gram negative forms, particularly *Pseudomonas*, has been demonstrated.[10] In the normal toe webs *C. minutissimum* is very commonly found without lesions yet erythrasma is a definite clinical entity. The reason a complex flora changes to permit a potentially pathogenic segment to cause lesions is usually unknown. Treatment enabling restoration of a normal flora often may be more effective than heroic antibacterial and antifungal treatment. Much more detailed study of microbial interactions is needed.[11,12]

Abnormal Conditions

Because the lower extremity is cool, moist and usually dirtier than the upper extremity, dermatophyte and atypical mycobacterial infections are common. The increased incidence of minor trauma often combined with poor vasculature makes secondary infection of traumatic lesions common. Poor vasculature can lead directly to stasis ulceration or gangrene with secondary colonization while neural involvement can produce similar lesions.

Frequently in lesions of the lower extremity, secondary microbial infections prolong and intensify the lesion and cause difficulty in diagnosis. The presence of a dermatophyte does not indicate tinea pedis or *S. aureus* a pyoderma. Conversely the ease with which significant colonization by these pathogens and *C. albicans*, *Pseudomonas* and *C. minutissimum* from the toe webs can occur must be recognized.

Experimental Approaches

It is clear that incidence data derived from group surveys are not the whole answer to the complex problem of microbially induced morbidity and its treatment. Quantitative techniques and detailed analysis of changes in the flora with treatment are in their infancy. However, the results of such studies are of practical value. Because examples of "athlete's foot" are readily available, detailed study of it can unravel both the pathogenesis of the various conditions lumped under this pseudodiagnosis as well as the activity of the various regimens prescribed.

References

1. Marples, M.J.: The Ecology of the Human Skin. Springfield, (Ill.), Charles C Thomas, 1965.
2. Pillsbury, D. M., and Rebell, G.: The bacterial flora of the skin. J. Invest. Derm., *18*:173, 1952.
3. Rebell, G., Pillsbury, D.M., de Saint Phalle, M., and Ginsburg, D.: Factors affecting the rapid disappearance of bacteria placed on the normal skin. J. Invest. Derm., *14*:247, 1950.
4. Marples, R.R.: The effect of hydration on the bacterial flora of the skin. *In* Maibach, H.I., and Hildick-Smith, G. (eds.): Skin Bacteria and Their Role in Infection. New York, McGraw-Hill, p. 33, 1965.
5. Marples, R.R.: Diphtheroids of normal human skin. Brit. J. Derm., *81* Suppl *1*:47, 1969.
6. Marples, M.J.: The Ecology of the Human Skin. Springfield, (Ill.), Charles C Thomas, 1965.
7. Rothmann, S.: Susceptibility factors in fungus infections in man. Trans. N.Y. Acad. Sci. Series II, *12*:27, 1949-1950.
8. Montes, L.F., and Wilborn, W.H.: Location of bacterial skin flora. Brit. J. Derm., *81* Suppl. *1*:23, 1969.
9. Marples, M.J., and Bailey, M.J.: A search for the presence of pathogenic bacteria and fungi in the interdigital spaces of the foot. Brit. J. Derm., *69*: 379, 1957.

10. Ehrenkrantz, N.J., Taplin, D., and Butt, P.: Antibiotic-resistant bacteria on the nose and skin: colonization and cross-infection. *In* Hobby, G. (ed.): Antimicrobial Agents and Chemotheraphy. Ann Arbor, American Society for Microbiology, 1967.

11. Sprunt, K., and Redman, W.: Evidence suggesting importance of role of enterobacterial inhibition in maintaining balance of normal flora. Ann. Intern. Med., *68*:579, 1968.

12. Marples, R.R., and Williamson, P.: Effects of systemic demethylchlortetracycline on human cutaneous microflora. Appl. Microbiol., *18*:228, 1969.

BACTERIAL INFECTIONS

The cutaneous bacterial infections, pyodermas and erythrasma, occur frequently on the lower extremities. Bacterial infections are often conveniently divided into primary and secondary pyodermas.

A primary infection originates in normal skin. Examples are impetigo, ecthyma, folliculitis, paronychia and erysipelas.

Secondary cutaneous infections occur on skin sites which are involved by a preceding dermatitis. Examples are infectious eczematoid dermatitis, infected intertrigo and ulcers with secondary infection.

PRIMARY PYODERMAS

Impetigo

Impetigo is a contagious, superficial skin infection which may be caused by staphylococci, or streptococci or both. Certain strains of staph or strep cause impetigo but rarely cause other types of skin lesions (Fig. 2-1).

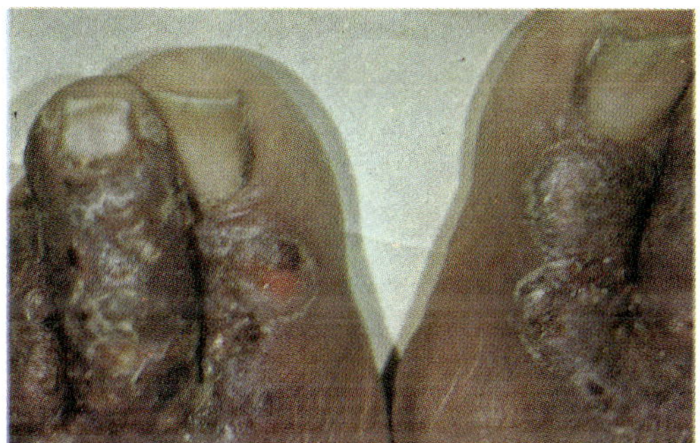

Fig. 2-1. Superficial pyoderma (impetigo).

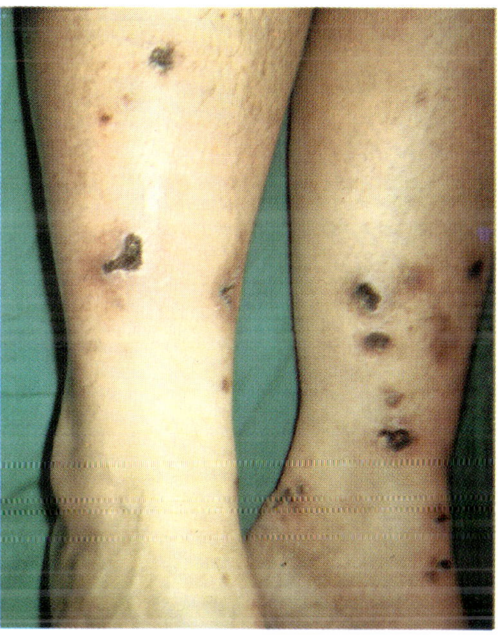

Fig. 2-2. Typical ecthyma. Group A streptococci recovered from lesions. A single injection of 600,000 units of benzathine penicillin G intramuscularly produced a rapid cure within a week.

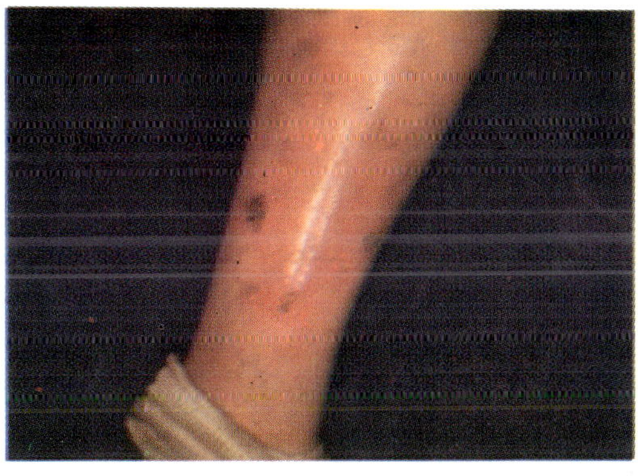

Fig. 2-3. Erysipelas of the leg. Demarcated, tense, inflamed plaque is characteristic. Systemic antibiotic (penicillin) is indicated.

Impetigo Contagiosa—usually affects grade-school children. It is quite contagious among infants but is less so among older children and adults. Clinically there are numerous thin-walled vesicles on an erythematous base which break readily and form yellowish crusts. Satellite lesions and peripheral extension may result in irregular serpiginous lesions. The crusts often become very thick and honey-colored with a "stuck-on" appearance. After they dry, they separate, leaving residual erythema but no scarring. Such lesions usually occur on the face, especially around the nose and mouth, but may occur anywhere on the skin except on the palms and soles. The lesions will resolve spontaneously in one or two weeks, more promptly with therapy, but occasionally may be prolonged.

Bullous Impetigo—a variant occuring in newborns and young children. Bullae appear which are less easily ruptured than the vesicles of impetigo contagiosa and tend to become larger. Eventually the bullae do rupture and form crusts. Peripheral extension occurs and large portions of the body may be involved, becoming crusted and denuded of skin.

Impetigo due to certain strains of streptococci may occasionally result in glomerulonephritis. In one series of patients with nephritis,[1] 33.8 percent had had a history of recent impetigo, though the experience of most clinicians would suggest that this percentage is higher than usually encountered.

A cornerstone of the therapy of impetigo is close attention to cleanliness with frequent washing of the lesions with an antibacterial soap. It is also essential that the crusts be removed by washing, compressing or gentle debridement. A topical antibiotic cream or ointment should be applied several times a day. Systemic antibiotics are not usually necessary but may occasionally be required if the impetigo is extensive or associated with lymphadenitis or fever. Nephritis reported following impetigo may be prevented by adequate systemic antibiotic administration.

Ecthyma

Ecthyma is a skin infection which begins as a small vesicle or pustule on an erythematous base. A hard adherent crust forms which can be difficult to remove. Under the crust a purulent irregular ulcer forms by extending into the dermis. Either staphylococci or streptococci may be cultured from the lesions. Healing occurs in a few weeks with scarring and hypo- or hyperpigmentation.

In temperate climates ecthyma usually occurs in children. In the tropics it is much more common and may affect any age. Lesions usually occur on the buttocks, thighs and legs (Fig. 2-2). Minor injuries often determine the site of the lesions. Treatment is similar to that for impetigo; however, systemic antibiotics are frequently indicated. Most effective is benzathine penicillin G; a single injection intramuscularly of 600,000 units will usually produce complete healing within a week. Since there is a tendency for recurrences, protective measures to prevent trauma are advisable.

Folliculitis

Folliculitis is a pyoderma occurring within a hair follicle. The lesion may be either superficial or deep. The extremities are a frequent location for superficial folliculitis. If the lesions are neglected, they may extend more deeply into the hair follicle and, in the beard or scalp areas, the infection may become chronic.

Occupational exposure to cutting oils and solvents may give rise to a folliculitis, though the pustules are usually sterile.

Paronychia

Paronychia is a cellulitis of the nail folds. Swelling, erythema, pain, tenderness and often a purulent discharge from beneath the nail fold occur. Secondary dystrophic changes of the nail are often seen. Frequent exposure of the digit to moisture, sweating, friction, maceration and systemic disorders, such as diabetes mellitus, will predispose to the development of paronychial infections and may cause acute infections to become chronic. In chronic paronychia, involvement with candida may occur.

Therapy consists of encouraging dryness and avoiding trauma to the nail fold, control of any underlying predisposing systemic disease, systemic antibiotics as indicated by culture and sensitivity tests. In addition, 2 percent or 4 percent thymol in chloroform applied by running a glass rod applicator along the edge of the nail fold several times daily will help maintain dryness and antibacterial activity under the separated nail fold. If a candida infection is present, specific topical antimonilial therapy (nystatin, amphotericin) should be instituted.

Erysipelas

Erysipelas is a streptococcal infection causing a sharply demarcated erythematous tense edematous plaque. Vesicles may be present in the advancing margin. The infection is usually acquired by direct inoculation into the skin and tends to occur in newborns, the elderly and others with lowered resistance. In adults, the leg is the site of involvement in 50 percent of the cases (Fig. 2-3).

Without therapy, complications (e.g., nephritis, subcutaneous abscesses and septicemia) are common, and in infants the mortality rate may reach 40 percent. Therapy with penicillin is effective. Recurrent attacks may lead to progressively severe lymphedema and the ultimate development of elephantiasis nostra verrucosa (see p. 186). At times low-dose prophylactic penicillin may be indicated to prevent recurrent attacks.

SECONDARY PYODERMAS

Infectious Eczematoid Dermatitis

Infectious eczematoid dermatitis is an eczematous inflammation resulting from the discharge of wet drainage seeping over the skin from an underlying cellulitis or pyogenic infection (Fig. 2-4). Autoinoculation often occurs. Therapy should be directed toward eradicating the primary site of infection. With control of the infection, the drainage ceases and the area of infectious eczematoid dermatitis clears.

Infected Intertrigo

Intertrigo is an inflammation of the skin resulting from the effects of friction, moisture and sweat retention. These factors also predispose to bacterial invasion and so it is not uncommon for some degree of bacterial infection to occur superimposed upon the intertrigo. Favorite sites of intertrigo are the axillae, crural regions, inframammary areas and between the toes, where it is often misdiagnosed as tinea (Fig. 2-5).

Treatment consists of promoting dryness of the intertriginous areas by ventilation, cool drying compresses and a bland, absorbent powder. The secondary infection is treated with the appropriate topical antibiotic in a lotion or compress form. Creams and ointments should be avoided.

Infected Ulcers

Ulcers of any etiology may become secondarily infected. Therapy consists of topical or systemic antibiotics and treatment of the underlying systemic or local cause of the ulcer itself. (See Chap. 8.)

Miscellaneous Pyogenic Infections

Rarely, may unusual organisms such as Pseudomonas and Proteus cause clinical pyodermic infections which are frequently resistant to the usual forms of antibacterial therapy. The causative organism and therapy should be determined by culture and sensitivities. Laboratory studies should be performed to determine the presence of any underlying systemic disorder such as diabetes, lymphoma or immunoglobulin defect, which would predispose to the establishment of a cutaneous infection by these uncommon invaders.

Figure 2-6 shows a recalcitrant pyoderma of the foot due to Pseudomonas which was resistant to the usual topical and systemic antibiotics and responded to acetic acid soaks, erythromycin ointment and Lassar's paste.

Erythrasma

For almost a century following its description, erythrasma was classified among the fungal disorders. However, in 1961, Sarkany and his coworkers[2,3] described the causative organism to be a gram positive bacillus and demonstrated that the clinical disease responded promptly to antibiotic therapy.

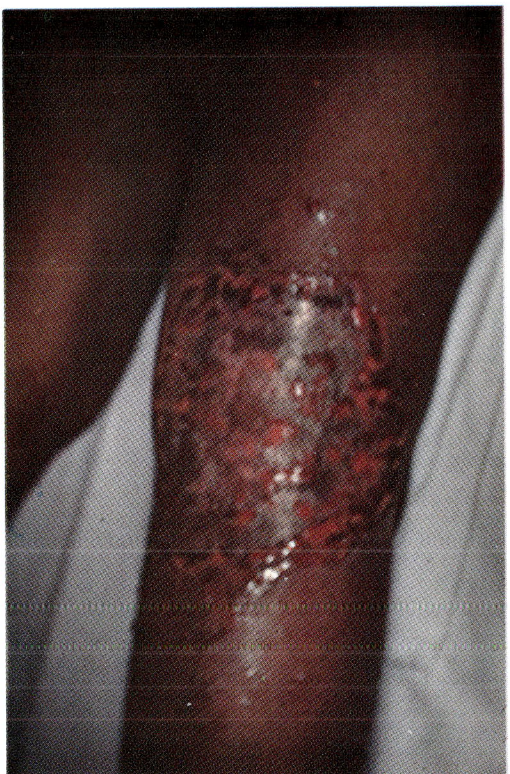

Fig. 2-4. Infectious eczematoid dermatitis secondary to underlying pyogenic infection. Therapy should be directed toward the pyogenic process; when the purulent drainage ceases, the dermatitis will clear.

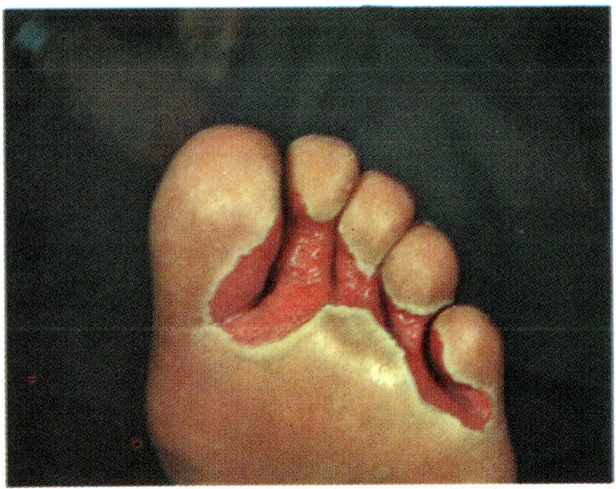

Fig. 2-5. Intertrigo with superimposed streptococcal infection. Frequently misdiagnosed as tinea pedis.

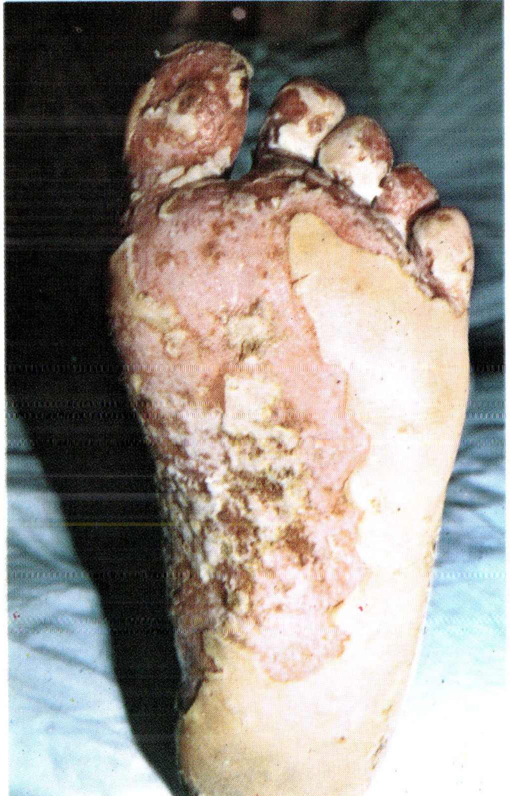

Fig. 2-6. Pseudomonas pyoderma. Systemic and local therapy were ineffective until acetic acid soaks were used. Laboratory studies did not reveal any underlying systemic disorder.

The lesions themselves are irregularly shaped, dry, scaly, well-demarcated patches showing a predilection for the crural folds, the pubic area, the axillae, intergluteal cleft, inframammary areas and the toe webs. The last mentioned location is the most common site of erythrasma and accounts for many of the instances of maceration and/or scaling, between the more lateral toes, which were not fungal in origin, or due to intertrigo and were not "white psoriasis."

If the diagnosis is suspected it is confirmed rather readily, since the lesions show a characteristic coral-red fluorescence under the Wood's light.[4] The organism *Corynebacterium minutissimum* can also be seen in scrapings stained with PAS or Giemsa. The organism can be cultured on special media the crucial ingredient of which is 20 percent fetal bovine serum, and the colonies will also produce the reddish fluorescence due to a porphyrin.

The use of erythromycin either locally or systemically results in dramatic disappearance of the skin eruption but recurrences may occur. Tetracycline is also effective.

The proper recognition of this entity may result in prompt resolution of a previously intractable and incapacitating intertrigo of the feet, as demonstrated in the two following case reports.

Case Report. A 77-year-old male was first hospitalized in July, 1968, for recurrent and recalcitrant erosions between the toes of both feet.

Examination revealed bilateral pedal atrophy and paresis as sequelae of childhood poliomyelitis with erosions and green purulent exudates between the toes of both feet. Fungal and bacterial cultures were unrewarding. Moderate improvement with Burow's soaks, 1:40, tetracycline 250 mg. p.o., q.i.d. and topical Castellani's paint was noted.

In October 1968, he was readmitted because of progression of the intertrigo and the development of an ulcer at the base of the left 3rd and 4th toes.

Examination revealed an absence of pulses below both femoral arteries, and a bruit over the left femoral artery, bilateral pedal edema, encrusted moist interdigital erosions and a mal perforans ulcer at the base of the left 3rd and 4th toes with gangrenous changes of the tip of the middle toe.

Wood's light examination revealed only a bright green fluorescence characteristic of Pseudomonas. Fungal studies were again nonproductive. Bacterial cultures of the erosion revealed Pseudomonas and Proteus species bilaterally.

Vasodilan 10 mg. q.i.d., penicillin G 400,000 units q.i.d., Burow's compresses, 1:40, acetic acid compresses 1/4 percent, Garamycin cream alternated with Lassar's paste resulted in moderate improvement over a 6-week hospitalization.

In January 1969, he was hospitalized for the third time within 6 months because of progression of the erosions and increased ischemic pain in the digit of the left foot.

Examination again revealed pedal edema, moist interdigital erosions with green crusts, gangrenous changes of the middle toes and a larger mal perforans. Fungal studies remained negative. Wood's light examination of the intertrigo revealed a coral-red fluorescence in several digital webs as well as the light green fluorescence of Pseudomonas. Bacterial cultures confirmed the presence of Pseudomonas species as well as a beta hemolytic Streptococcus Group A (Fig. 2-7).

Therapy with erythromycin 250 mg. p.o., q.i.d., Vasodilan 10 mg. q.i.d., skim-milk compresses and chloramphenical cream was instituted.

After 14 days, pedal edema resolved, the erosions and mal perforans healed and ischemic pain could be controlled by occasional Darvon, 65 mg., capsules (Fig. 2-8).

Follow-up Wood's light examination failed to reveal either erythrasma or Pseudomonas.

Comment. The rapid response of an otherwise debilitating and recalcitrant problem of intertrigo of the toes, complicated by obliterative vascular disease was based upon two factors. The underlying cause of the intertrigo, erythrasma, was finally appreciated and treated with erythromycin. Previously the luxurious overgrowth of Pseudomonas and other opportunistic pathogens obscured the presence of erythrasma.

Case Report. A 74-year-old male developed an eczematous eruption of his feet, most marked in the interdigital spaces of his toes. Allergic contact dermatitis was ruled out by appropriate patch testing. Attempts to culture a fungus were repeatedly unsuccessful. Moderate improvement of the eruption was obtained after several months of therapy consisting of systemic tetracycline, Burow's compresses and elevation of the feet.

A year later, because of an exacerbation of the intertrigo that was unresponsive to potassium permanganate compresses, griseofulvin systemically, Castellani's paint and Whitfield's ointment, a Wood's lamp examination of the interdigital spaces was performed. The typical coral-red fluorescence of erythrasma was noted between most of the affected toes.

An attempt to grow *C. minutissimum* on special media was unsuccessful, due to the heavy growth of Proteus species and lactose fermenting gram-negative bacilli. Although all organisms were resistant to erythromycin, therapy consisting of erythromycin 250 mg. q.i.d., skim-milk compresses, and chloramphenical cream topically, was instituted. The intertrigo cleared in 2 weeks.

SYSTEMIC BACTERIAL INFECTIONS

A variety of bacterial infections may cause lesions of the skin and also have the potentiality for systemic involvement. Examples are diphtheria, anthrax, erysipeloid, brucellosis, tularemia, tuberculosis, syphilis and leprosy.

The majority of these disorders show no predilection for the lower extremities and are therefore not reviewed. Erythema induratum is discussed under the nodose lesions (Chap. 7); the lesions of syphilis are under a separate section of this chapter.

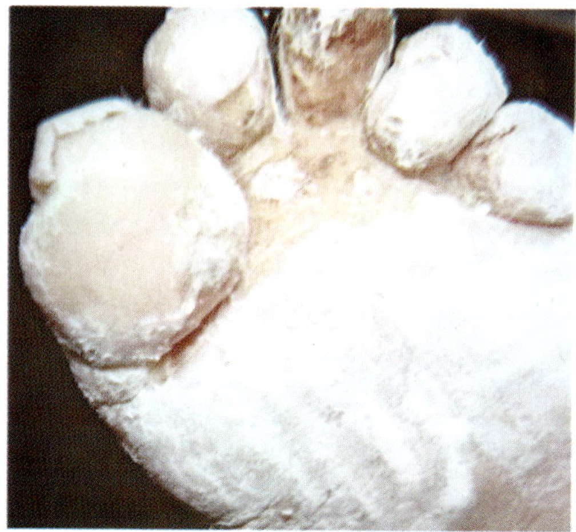

Fig. 2-7. Erythrasma with superimposed Pseudomonas infection.

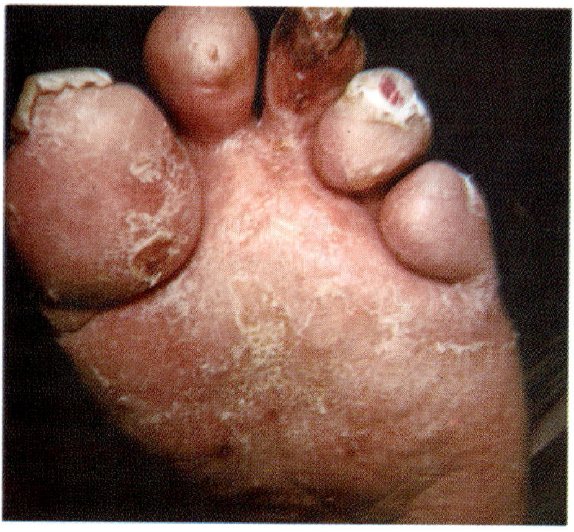

Fig. 2-8. Appearance of foot of same patient following treatment with erythromycin for erythrasma.

References

1. McCullough, G. C. *et al.*: Acute glomerulonephritis: impetigo as an etiological factor. J. Pediat., *38*:346, 1951.

2. Sarkany, I., Taplin, D., and Blank, H.: Erythrasma – common bacterial infection of the skin. JAMA, *177*:130, 1961.

3. Sarkany, I. Taplin, D., and Blank, H.: The etiology and treatment of erythrasma. J. Invest. Derm., *37*:283, 1961.

4. Michaelides, P., and Shatin, H.: Erythrasma fluorescence under the Wood light. Arch. Derm. Syph., *65*:614, 1952.

FUNGAL INFECTIONS

The fungi which affect man are relatively few, and their effect is often rather benign. But they may also cause severe, even fatal, diseases.

The feet are particularly susceptible to the geophilic (soil-dwelling) fungi, especially in warmer climates where the feet are often bare. The legs and feet are also likely to come in contact with animals and their zoophilic fungi. In addition, the anthropophilic fungi are quite opportunistic and often find ideal conditions existing on the feet—warmth and moisture due to the occlusion of shoes, intertriginous maceration between the toes, moist hyperkeratosis of the soles and the effects of aging, trauma and vascular disease.

Since human beings are constantly exposed to fungal elements throughout most, if not all, of their lives, clinical dermatomycotic infections would seem virtually unavoidable. Yet, in fact, such widespread infection does not occur because of wide variation in individual resistance and susceptibility. In some fungus infections (*T. mentagrophytes*) there appears to be a fluctuation or alternation in immunity and susceptibility; an individual low rate of physiological desquamation may play a role in *T. rubrum* infection. Severe systemic or debilitating diseases may markedly influence the course of a *T. rubrum* infection.

The means by which fungal infections are acquired and transmitted are not entirely known. Some investigators favor the theory that dermatophyte infections are acquired from fungi dispersed in the environment. Causal organisms have been isolated from footwear, locker room floors, shower stalls, foot baths and swimming pool areas; in some studies, the percentage of infected individuals was correlated with the frequency with which swimming pools or bathing environment were cleaned. However, other investigators feel that this epidemiologic evidence is circumstantial. Rosenthal *et al.*[1] were unable to isolate pathogenic fungi from shower room floors, locker rooms and swimming pools. They also found it extremely difficult to experimentally infect volunteers whose feet were immersed in foot baths containing heavy inocula of fungi. No clinical infections could be produced in 68 such volunteers. The one way they were able to establish infection was by inducing blister formation prior to immersion in the contaminated foot bath. They concluded that exogenous exposure to fungi plays a minor role in infection; rather it is decreased local resistance of the skin which accounts for the activation of infection by endogenous fungi. Support for this concept are the studies of Strauss and Kligman[2] who found that the soles and nails were the stable reservoirs of fungi and served as chief sources of acute attacks of interdigital tinea pedis.

Frequent bathing decreases the chance of infection by removing a significant quantity of the infectious material and also by decreasing the amount of organic residues of perspiration on which some fungi feed. Skin which is naturally thin, with little keratin, is more difficult to infect. Oily, moist skin is more readily infected than dry skin which desquamates more readily. Normal human serum contains a fungistatic agent which diffuses through the tissue and keeps the fungal infection superficial.

It is also clear that many people are completely resistant to infection by some fungi. An example is the commonly observed situation in which a husband or wife will have a chronic *T. rubrum* infection of the feet for many years while the spouse remains totally free of infection.

Tinea pedis, the most common of the dermatomycoses, is usually due to *Trichophyton rubrum* or *Trichophyton mentagrophytes*, with *Epidermophyton floccosum* a less frequent causative organism.

The manifestations of tinea pedis vary widely but generally consist of two main clinical pictures: the acute inflammatory and chronic hyperkeratotic types.

ACUTE INFLAMMATORY TINEA PEDIS

In this form of fungal infection, the skin is involved with an oozing, macerated, vesicular eruption which leads to the loss of the epidermis, fissuring, pruritus and occasionally secondary bacterial infection. Frequently, the initial area of involvement is in a toe web, usually the 4th interspace (Fig. 2-9), where maceration and fissuring occur. The process may then extend to other toe webs and may involve large areas of the sole (Fig. 2-10). *Trichophyton mentagrophytes* is the usual causative fungus in acute inflammatory tinea pedis with *Epidermophyton floccosum* the etiologic agent less frequently.

CHRONIC HYPERKERATOTIC TINEA PEDIS

In marked contrast to the acute vesicular inflammatory tinea pedis is the exceedingly chronic scaling, often asymptomatic, hyperkeratotic type. In this disorder, the involvement is on the soles often extending onto the sides of the feet, the so-called moccasin distribution (Fig. 2-11). The toe webs are usually spared. This type of tinea pedis is almost always due to *Trichophyton rubrum*.

A peculiarity of chronic *T. rubrum* infections is their occasional tendency to persist as an asymmetric disorder. Only one foot may be involved for many years and when the hands as well as the feet are involved, almost invariably only a single hand will be infected. The explanation for this behavior is unknown and is not related to the patient's being right- or left-handed.

Perifollicular granulomas (Majocchi's) caused by penetration of hairs infected with *T. rubrum* through breaks in the follicular wall are occasionally seen on the lower legs (Fig. 2-12).

Fungal infection of the toenails (onychomycosis) (Fig. 2-13) may be the only manifestation of tinea pedis or may be present along with cutaneous involvement of the feet. The infection begins at the distal tip of the nail and slowly spreads proximally resulting in opaque yellowish discoloration, crumbling and distortion of the nail with accumulation of soft subungual hyperkeratotic debris.

Dermatophytid or id reactions (Fig. 2-14) are secondary eruptions occurring on the fingers and hands of sensitized individuals as a result of the spread of fungi or their allergenic products from a primary site. Id reactions can also occur on the feet and legs. The lesions usually present as tense discrete pruritic vesicles. They are seen in *T. mentagrophytes* infections which have been irritated or overtreated. Fungi can be found in the primary lesion, but the secondary id lesion is sterile. The id lesions involute with the clearing of the primary focus; patients respond positively to skin tests with trichophytin.

While fungal infections are among the most frequent skin affections of the feet, many nonfungal disorders are misdiagnosed as tinea pedis (e.g., intertrigo, erythrasma, contact dermatitis, dyshidrosis, neurodermatitis and psoriasis appearing as marginated hyperkeratotic plaques, as "white" psoriasis of toe webs, or as pustular psoriasis). Tinea actually accounts for only about one-third of skin disease involving the feet. Onychomycosis must be differentiated from nail changes occurring in psoriasis, lichen planus and alopecia areata, and as the result of recurrent paronychial infections and trauma. All clinical diagnoses of fungus infection of the feet should be confirmed by laboratory studies.

Diagnosis

The laboratory confirmation of tinea pedis and tinea unguium is relatively easy and should be carried out in all suspected cases. There are two basic techniques, the direct microscopic examination of samples of diseased skin for fungal elements and fungal culture.

Examination of skin scrapings: Sponge the surface of the affected skin with 70 percent alcohol, let it dry, and then with a No. 15 bladed scalpel, scrape small portions of involved tissue. It is advisable to take material from the more active portions of the lesions and to scrape deep enough to cause minimal bleeding. Place the flakes of keratin on a clean slide or implant onto culture media. If the skin is blistered, clip the top of a vesicle and place it inverted on a glass slide. In nail infection, scrape away the loose surface debris and take material from well under the nails. Add a drop or two of 10 percent potassium hydroxide, apply a cover slip and gently heat the slide (over a Bunsen flame, alcohol lamp, or by placing on the lid of a heated sterilizer) for a few seconds to facilitate digestion of keratin. Examine the slide under low power with subdued light. Fungal elements appear as branching, threadlike hyphae about 2 to 4 microns in diameter, somewhat double-walled and sometimes showing cross walls. If the first specimen proves negative, repeat the examination with material from other areas of the lesion.

At times it may be difficult to detect hyphae among epithelial cells and other debris, even with potassium hydroxide digestion, particularly since there are no color differences. Recently a new rapid contrast stain has been reported[3] greatly facilitating the reading of such microscopic preparations. The contrast stain consists of two solutions: (1) one part 1 percent aerosol OTB, one part 10 percent potassium hydroxide, and 2 parts 1 percent ink blue P.P.; and (2) 0.5 percent rose bengal in buffered Shear's mounting fluid. Using this stain, on direct

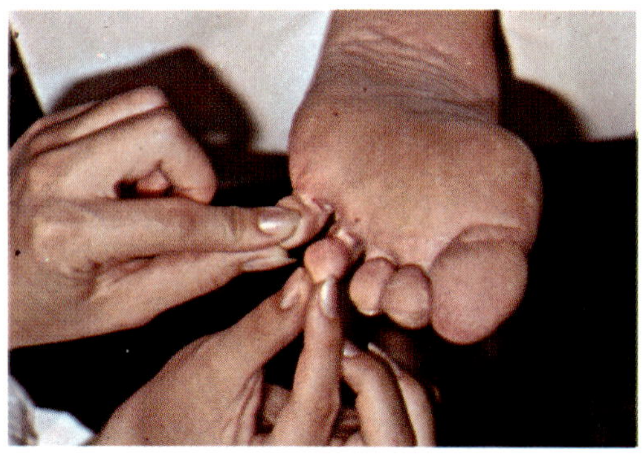

Fig. 2-9. Interdigital fungal infection characteristic of *T. mentagrophytes.*

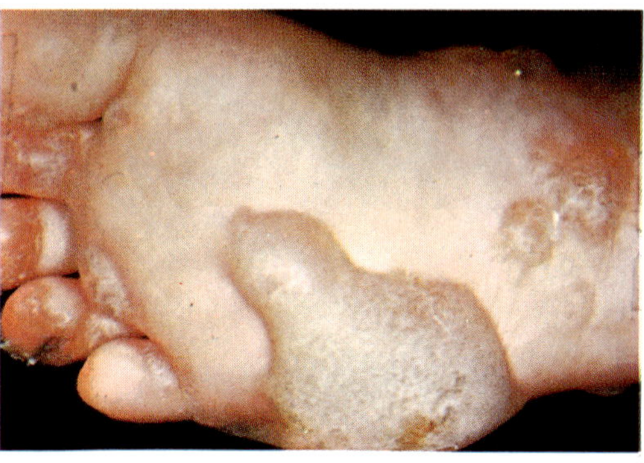

Fig. 2-10. Tinea pedis. Severe vesiculobullous reaction. *T. mentagrophytes* cultured.

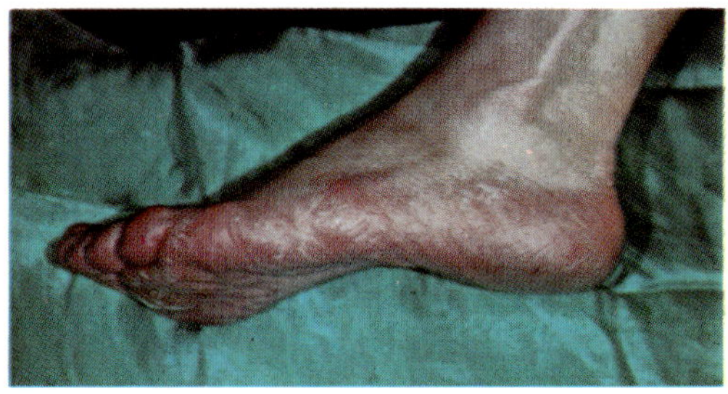

Fig. 2-11. *T. rubrum* of foot—characteristic moccasin distribution.

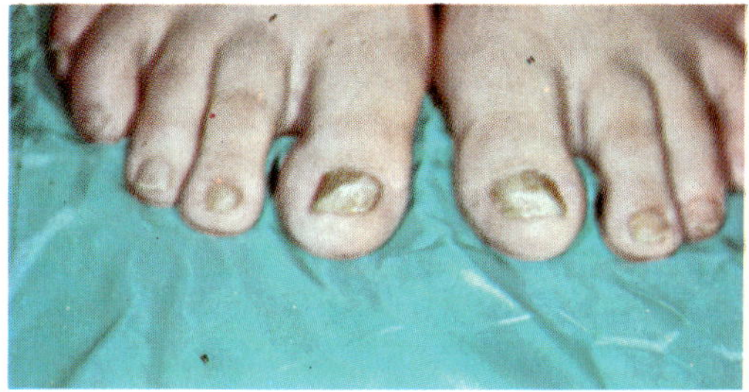

Fig. 2-13. Onychomycosis (*T. rubrum*).

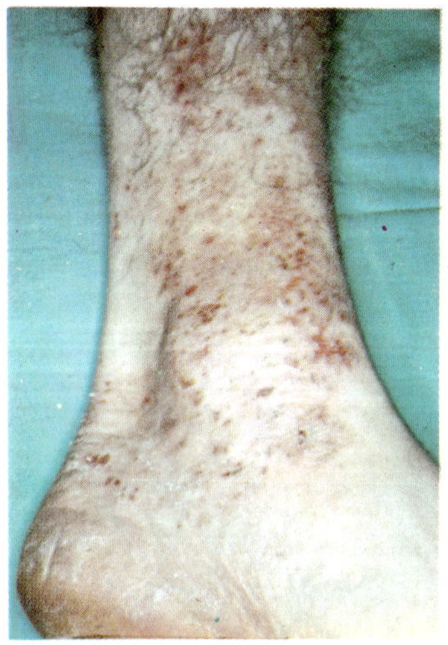

Fig. 2-12. Majocchi's granuloma (*T. rubrum*). The follicular inflamed papules are characteristic.

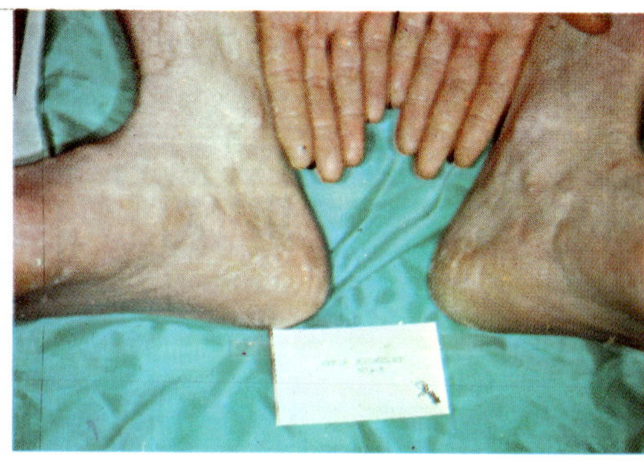

Fig. 2-14. Tinea pedis (*T. mentagrophytes*) with trichophytid.

microscopic examination of scrapings, dermatophyte hyphae stain light blue against a background of rose-red keratinocytes. Candida hyphae and pseudohyphae stain blue; cytoplasm of blastospores stains pink, the walls blue. The background is rose-red. Geotrichum, Trichosporon and Aspergillus stain similarly.

Scrapings may also be placed on Sabouraud's agar and incubated at room temperature for from 2 to 6 weeks. If growth occurs, this not only confirms the clinical diagnosis but allows identification of the organism.

Recently Taplin *et al.*[4] developed a fungal culture medium allowing identification of dermatophytes by simple observation of a color change of the medium. The medium contains phenol red which is yellow at the acid pH of the agar. The dermatophytes produce alkaline metabolites that raise the pH of the medium and result in changing phenol red from yellow to red. This striking color change does not occur with saprophytes or with most candida strains. The agar contains additives that inhibit the growth of bacterial organisms. Experience both in the United States and Vietnam has shown this new medium to be at least 97 percent reliable. Nail scrapings containing large amounts of saprophytic fungi may give a false positive color change; for this reason the new medium is not recommended for identification of dermatophytes from nails. An occasional strain of *Candida albicans* may produce the red color. The caps on the culture tubes should be kept loose, since false negative reactions may occur if the caps are tightly closed. Cultures should be read within 14 days to decrease the chance of eventual growth of extraneous organisms producing false reactions.

Since the dermatophytes show the characteristic agar color change and are responsive to griseofulvin, the color change medium allows easy differentiation of those fungi that will respond to griseofulvin from those that will not. The medium is available commercially as the Pfizer Dermatophyte Test Medium (DTM).

Treatment

Acute Inflammatory Exacerbations. For acute inflammatory exacerbations with secondary eczematization, use mild therapy to control the dermatitis first and treat the fungous disease later.

External measures:

Soaks or wet compresses for 20 minutes, 3 or 4 times daily.
Apply bland topical preparations as Burow's paste between soaks.
Topical antibiotics may be used if secondary infection is present.
Rest, partial or complete; feet should be kept elevated if edema is present.
Open shoes or sandals if patient is ambulatory.
Avoid fungicidal chemicals during this stage; they are often too irritating for eczematous areas and may cause id reactions.

Internal measures:

When cellulitis and/or lymphangitis are present, use broad-spectrum antibiotics.
For severe forms of eczematization, oral corticosteroids may be indicated.

Subacute, Chronic or Mild Infections. For subacute, chronic or mild infections, do the following:

External measures:

Use powders, tinctures or solutions during the day. Tolnaftate is very effective.
Antifungal creams or ointments are prescribed for night use.

We give our patients a list of instructions to follow:
Directions for care of feet

1. Soak feet in solution prescribed, morning and evening and before retiring.
2. Dry your feet well.
3. Change socks twice daily, morning and evening. Socks should be cotton; avoid synthetic materials.
4. Change shoes twice daily, morning and evening.
5. Powder well, your feet, socks and shoes, twice daily.
6. Apply medicine given every night as directed.

Internal measures:

Griseofulvin has revolutionized the therapy of fungal infections but it is not without its drawbacks. The drug is fungistatic, not fungicidal. It operates by becoming incorporated in the keratin layer as it is formed and inhibits the fungus until the organisms are shed with the keratin. Treatment with griseofulvin must be continued for 3 or 4 weeks in skin infections and from 6 months to one year or longer in onychomycosis. The dose of griseofulvin is 250 to 500 mg. daily of the micronized type. Some persons require 1000 mg., particularly those with chronic nail infections. The necessity of long-term treatment in onychomycosis should be stressed to the patient; "trials" of 3 to 4 months usually end up as disappointing treatment failures. It has been shown that intestinal absorption is enhanced by taking the griseofulvin after a fatty meal. Tinea pedis and onychomycosis may be persistent and recurrent in spite of therapy with griseofulvin or topical agents. Because of the problem of constant reinfection, the cure rate in onychomycosis is only 60 to 70 percent despite vigorous therapy.

Side effects from griseofulvin include gastrointestinal distress, loose stools, headaches, urticarial and morbilliform eruptions. In some patients, griseofulvin, particularly in high doses, may cause slowing of reaction time and interference with coordinated movements. The drug should therefore be administered with caution to airplane pilots and auto drivers. In rare instances griseofulvin may cause hematologic alterations ranging from leukopenia to an L.E. syndrome, and by enzymatic interference may induce porphyria.

Some clinicians advocate evulsion of the nails in chronic onychomycosis. In our experience we have found this to be of no value.

FUNGAL INFECTIONS IN COMBAT TROOPS IN VIETNAM

The importance of moisture in increasing the extent and persistence of dermatophyte infections has been graphically demonstrated among the combat troops in Vietnam.[5] In the humid tropical environment, spending many hours in water with little or no opportunity to dry out, bathe or put on clean dry clothes, skin problems have incapacitated as many as 25 to 40 percent of combat personnel, with fungous infections and tropical acne the major causes.

The most frequent dermatophytosis was a *Trichophyton mentagrophytes* infection which, in the damp environment, frequently extended beyond the anticipated areas of involvement, such as the feet and crural areas, to cover widespread areas of the body surface. Frequently dermatophyte involvement of the leg corresponding to the upper portion of the combat boots was as intense as the involvement of the feet. The widespread lesions often took the form of an inflammatory folliculitis.

The organisms cultured and tested were sensitive to griseofulvin and one would anticipate a good response to this therapy. However, it was frequently impractical for men in the field to take an adequate dose for the necessary length of time.

References

1. Rosenthal, S.A. *et al.*: Studies on the dissemination of fungi from the feet of subjects with and without fungous disease of the feet. J. Invest. Derm., *26*:41, 1956.

2. Strauss, J.S., and Kligman, A.M.: An experimental study of tinea pedis and onychomycosis of the foot. Arch. Derm., *76*:70, 1957.

3. Swartz, J.H., and Medrek, T.F.: Rapid contrast stain as a diagnostic aid for fungous infections. Arch. Derm., *99*:494, 1969.

4. Taplin, D., Zaias, N., Rebell, G., and Blank, H.: Isolation and recognition of dermatophytes on a new medium (DTM). Arch. Derm., *99*:203, Feb., 1969.

5. Blank, H., Taplin, D., and Zaias, N.: Cutaneous *Trichophyton Mentagrophytes* infections in Vietnam. Arch. Derm., 99:135, 1969.

CANDIDIASIS

Candidiasis, or moniliasis, is separated from the dermatophytes because it is caused by a quite different fungus. *Candida albicans* is a yeastlike fungus, occurring as a normal inhabitant of the gastrointestinal tract. Normal persons with normal skin are fairly resistant. It is rather an adventitious pathogen and exerts its influence as a disease-producer in altered physiologic states, such as prolonged or massive antibiotic therapy, diabetes, alcoholism, obesity, vascular stasis, excessive moisture, vitamin deficiencies, or states of abnormal proteinemia. While monilial infections are usually superficial, a generalized or systemic infection occasionally will occur in the presence of a predisposing systemic disorder. On the lower extremities candidiasis may manifest itself as interdigital and intertriginous infections, paronychia and onycholysis, and monilial granuloma.

Intertrigo may occur wherever two skin surfaces are opposed to each other, thereby preventing adequate ventilation and evaporation of sweat. Intertrigo may occur between the toes of those persons who have thick, stubby, tightly opposed toes or in persons with normal shaped toes but who wear tight shoes and occlusive socks preventing adequate evaporation in warm weather. The candida infection gives rise to white, macerated tissue with fissuring and denuded areas, particularly in the fourth interdigital space, and is known as erosio interdigitalis blastomycetica.[1]

Paronychia and onycholysis commonly are produced by candida infections of the fingernails, but occasional involvement of the toenails occurs. The tissue adjacent to and including the nail fold becomes red, edematous and tender. The posterior nail fold is raised from the underlying nail and the nail becomes opaque and dystrophic. Harboring of moisture in this sulcus leads to further progression of the monilial infection. There may be further involvement distally separating the nail bed from the overlying plate, possibly giving the nail the appearance of being depressed proximally and elevated distally. Only one nail may be involved, but more often several or all are affected.

A rare form of cutaneous candidiasis seen on the feet, as well as on the hands, face or scalp, is the monilial granuloma. This is a generalized or disseminate form of the disease, and is characterized by multiple nodules which may break down to form fungating, granulomatous tissue with overlying crusting due to the oozing.[2]

The laboratory diagnosis of candidiasis is usually rather readily made. A potassium hydroxide preparation, as previously described, will show yeastlike budding forms. Culture of the organism yields a soft, white, shiny colony which grows much more rapidly than the dermatophytes. However, since monilial organisms are present on normal skin and only a few such yeast forms are necessary to yield a positive culture, the recovery of monilia on Sabouraud's agar does not constitute proof of a significant fungus infection. Only when the KOH slide preparation shows the typical yeastlike budding forms can the diagnosis of candidiasis be accepted.

Treatment of monilial intertrigo consists basically of bringing about and maintaining a dry environment through drying compresses, Castellani's paint and proper aeration. Topical preparations of nystatin (Mycostatin), amphotericin B (Fungizone) or vioform are of benefit; candida is unaffected by griseofulvin. Candida paronychia or onycholysis respond well to maintenance of a dry environment and topical application of a solution of 4 percent thymol in chloroform applied to the gap between the posterior nail fold and the nail plate twice daily. Cut away the free edge of the nail involved in onycholysis to allow adequate drying and exposure of the nail bed to the same thymol in chloroform medication. Monilial granuloma requires therapy with systemic amphotericin B.

In generalized or disseminate forms of candidiasis, as well as those localized infections peculiarly resistant or recurrent, it is obligatory to suspect and search for underlying metabolic or physiologic derangements that may predispose to candidiasis.

References

1. Wilson, J.W., and Plunkett, O.A.: The Fungous Diseases of Man. p. 168. University of California Press, 1965.

2. Hauser, F.V., and Rothman, S.: Monilial granuloma. Arch. Derm. and Syph., *61*: 297, 1950.

DEEP FUNGAL INFECTIONS

In contrast to the dermatophytes producing primarily superficial infections, there are a group of pathogenic fungi that thrive in the deeper tissue and viscera, having the potential to produce systemic disease. They may become manifest on the lower extremities and are acquired either by inhalation, ingestion or inoculation. Occasionally the disease, though acquired by way of the respiratory or gastrointestinal tract, may disseminate systemically and may manifest itself on the skin. If the infection is acquired by inoculation, it may involve more critical structures by direct extension, lymphatic spread, or dissemination by the blood stream.

Coccidioidomycosis. It is a deep fungal infection caused by the organism *Coccidioides immitis* and is usually contracted in the southwestern United States, and parts of Mexico and Central America, by inhalation of the spores of *Coccidioides immitis* in the dusty soil. The most common form of infection is a pneumonia-like disease which often is subclinical or mildly limited. However, in rare instances it may become disseminated and produce clinical manifestations in the bones, central nervous system, or skin. On the lower extremities the skin lesions may present as chronic abscesses or granulomas of a pustular, erosive, ulcerative, warty, or vegetating type which frequently are significantly secondarily infected. This disseminated form of coccidioidomycosis represents an inability of the individual to handle his disease immunologically, and carries a grave prognosis.

Another recently described, though very rare, form of coccidioidomycosis is the chancriform or primary inoculation type, often appearing in the lower extremities due to contact with contaminated soil. The lesion is a painless, indurated nodule or plaque with central ulceration possibly accompanied by lymphadenopathy or nodules along the lymphatics. These lesions almost always heal within a few weeks with no treatment. If the lesion persists for months, it is unlikely that it arose by primary cutaneous inoculation.

The diagnosis of coccidioidomycosis may be made by demonstrating the organism in pus or biopsy material, but more definitively by culturing the organism. The coccidioidin skin test usually becomes positive 3 or 4 weeks after infection, and remains positive for many years, perhaps for life. A false negative reaction may be noted in overwhelming disease. The complement fixation test is also helpful in making the diagnosis and in following the results of treatment.

Coccidioides immitis is susceptible to the antifungal agent, amphotericin B. This is the treatment of choice in generalized infections. On the lower extremities abscesses may require excision or drainage in conjunction with systemic therapy.

Histoplasmosis. This is one of the most common systemic fungal infections. Usually the disease is pulmonary, though it may become disseminate; cutaneous manifestations on the lower extremities are fairly rare. *Histoplasma capsulatum*, the causative organism, is found most frequently in North America, particularly in the North Central

United States along the Mississippi and its tributaries and is mainly acquired by inhalation of dust. There is apparently a relationship between infected soil and excreta from some birds and poultry.

The skin lesions of disseminate histoplasmosis are similar to the lesions of coccidioidomycosis, though occurring much less frequently on the lower extremities. Mucous membrane lesions are not uncommon and may present as either ulcers or granulomatous masses. A rare primary cutaneous form of histoplasmosis acquired by direct inoculation presents as a chancriform lesion and follows a course similar to that described for coccidioidomycosis.

The diagnosis of histoplasmosis may be made by demonstrating the organism in the pus from cutaneous lesions, or by cultures on Sabouraud's agar at body or room temperature. The histoplasmin skin test is a reliable aid to diagnosis and once positive remains so for several years. In severe systemic histoplasmosis, the skin test may be negative. The complement-fixation test has diagnostic and prognostic significance; a rising titer indicates a poor prognosis. A precipitin test is also available which correlates with 83 percent accuracy with the complement-fixation test.

Amphotericin B given intravenously is the treatment of choice for histoplasmosis.

Sporotrichosis. This is a deep fungal infection in which the lesions are manifested most frequently on the skin. The causative fungus *Sporotrichum schenckii* is found in soil and on many forms of vegetation. The disease thus is seen most frequently among farmers, gardeners, florists or outdoor laborers. Approximately 60 percent of lesions occur on the hand or arm, 23 percent on the trunk, 11 percent on the legs. The organism must be inoculated into the subcutaneous tissue through a break in the skin, or through contamination of an open sore or wound.

The primary lesion begins days or weeks after contact and consists of a painless, enlarging papule that forms an ulcerated, indurated lesion. After a week or more, the ulcer is followed by a series of erythematous, firm, painless nodules along the lymphatic chain draining the area, which may also break down to form ulcers. Lymphangitis is present and the regional lymph nodes become enlarged, but usually do not ulcerate. In general, the patient's health is not affected, but the localized lesions rarely heal spontaneously. In some cases the lymphatic involvement may be minimal or even absent completely, and the primary lesion spreads in the skin itself forming an erythematous flat plaque, either smooth or covered with silvery scales. When occurring on the knees, the lesion may take on a warty form sometimes with associated pustulation.

A disseminated form of sporotrichosis may exist when hematogenous spread gives rise to multiple subcutaneous nodular masses over the skin anywhere on the body. These soften and break down also to form chronic ulcerations.

It has been postulated that the organisms may be inhaled or ingested to give rise to infections of the respiratory or gastrointestinal tract, the so-called nontegumentary primary sporotrichosis. It has not been convincingly shown that this form of infection does in fact exist.

Sporotrichum schenkii is almost impossible to diagnose on histological examination of the lesions and the foremost necessity in diagnosis is the culture of the organism on Sabouraud's agar from the suspect lesion. Skin and serologic tests exist but there is some uncertainty as to their reliability and to the proper interpretation of test results.

The disease responds remarkably to treatment with saturated solution of potassium iodide; 15 drops in milk or water 3 times a day is usually effective. Therapy must be carried out until the lesion involutes and then at least 4 to 6 weeks after apparent clinical cure.

Chromoblastomycosis (Chromomycosis). This uncommon "deep" fungal infection, confined entirely to the skin, has been associated with certain fungi of the genus *Phialophora.* These are soil-dwelling organisms in all parts of the world. The distribution of the disease, however, is predominantly among barefooted farm laborers in the tropics. The majority of cases occur on the feet or legs below the knees, supporting the theory of inoculation from the soil. Occasionally lesions occur on areas of the body that are normally clothed and it has been postulated that these cases represent instances of cutaneous dissemination from a previously unrecognized primary focus in the lungs.

The initial lesion is a papule or pustule persisting unchanged for a prolonged period and then enlarging and ulcerating. Verrucous fungating lesions eventually develop which enlarge by peripheral extension with irregular central clearing and atrophic scar formation (Fig. 2-15). The lesions are often involved by secondary bacterial infection which in turn may lead to lymphatic stasis and elephantiasis.

Systemic therapy for chromoblastomycosis is difficult and uncertain, since all the fungi involved are resistant to amphotericin B. Oral potassium iodide and calciferol or local perfusion with amphotericin B have occasionally resulted in apparent cures. Local treatment consists of excision of the involved area with primary closure or grafting. Marked extension with debilitation of the individual has occasionally required amputation.

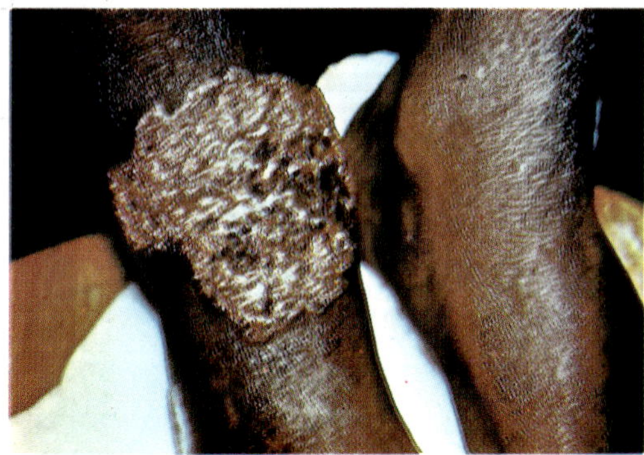

Fig. 2-15. Chromoblastomycosis. Typical verrucous, fungating lesion.

Blastomycosis. This is a deep fungal infection due to *Blastomyces dermatitidis*, which at times may be confused with chromoblastomycosis. In most cases the organism is probably inhaled as a dust, causing a primary pulmonary focus which usually is subclinical but occasionally may give rise to cutaneous lesions by dissemination.

Primary cutaneous blastomycosis, an extremely rare form of the disease, occurs apparently by inoculation directly into the foot or leg. Clinically it resembles sporotrichosis including the lymphatic involvement.

The most common form is the chronic cutaneous type, probably caused by hematogenous dissemination from a fleeting or subclinical primary pulmonary blastomycosis. Other organs may be involved in the disseminated form, but it is the skin which is most often and primarily involved. The disease starts as an isolated erythematous papule or subcutaneous nodule that ruptures to form an ulcer, crusts over and spreads peripherally, eventually forming an elevated plaque. On close inspection, the margin of the lesion abruptly falls off to meet normal tissue and the surface of the plaque may be studded with minute abscesses. Ulcers, subcutaneous abscesses or sinus tracts may form. The central area of the plaque may clear spontaneously, giving rise to a circinate lesion with a highly active serpiginous border.

The organism may be found on microscopic examination of pus or serous fluid as single budding yeast forms. Culture of the organism is readily obtained at either room or body temperatures. The blastomycin skin test and the complement-fixation test are of less diagnostic value than for histoplasmosis.

The treatment of choice is intravenous amphotericin B to which the fungus is sensitive. Well-localized lesions on the lower extremities may

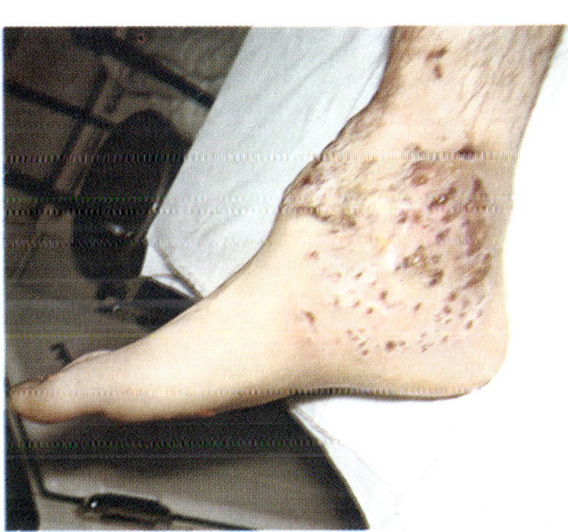

Fig. 2-16. Mycetoma (*N. brasiliensis*) before treatment. The granulomatous lesion contains multiple draining sinuses.

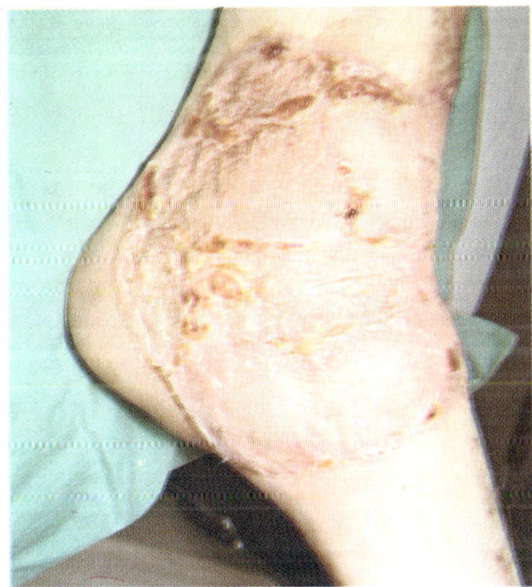

Fig. 2-17. Mycetoma (following excision and split-thickness skin graft. Patient also received sulfadiazine therapy).

be excised. However, occult dissemination to other organs may be present. Excision must be accompanied by systemic therapy with amphotericin B.

Mycetoma. This deep fungus infection, limited almost exclusively to the realm of the lower extremities, is mycetoma (Madura foot or maduromycosis). Mycetoma is a general term meaning any tumor produced by fungi; the term maduromycosis should be used only for mycetoma due to filamentous fungi and not from the bacteria-like actinomycetes. The disease is concentrated in scattered regions of the tropics and subtropics including Mexico, Guatemala and South America and may be caused by several organisms including the actinomycetes group (*Actinomyces israelii*, *Nocardia* sp., *Streptomyces* sp.) and the true fungi (*Allescheria boydii*, *Cephalosporium* sp., *Madurella* sp., *Phialophora* sp.).

The mode of infection is inoculation of the involved organism through the plantar skin, aided by the fact that, in the tropics, plantation workers, workers in rice paddies, or natives, for pure comfort or lack of footwear, go barefooted throughout life. At the site of inoculation there arises a painless, indurated nodule which enlarges indolently and breaks down to form granulation tissue and sinuses which exude pus containing tiny granules of varying colors. These granules are minute clumps of the fungus being extruded by the tissues. More nodules appear in adjacent areas and connecting sinuses are formed. Through fusion of these lesions, the involved area may encompass a whole foot and part of the leg with tremendous swelling, hypertrophy and multiple sinuses (Fig. 2-16). Some of the sinuses extend to the bone and osteomyelitis may be extensive and quite destructive. The foot may become so massive as to prohibit its use, and its owner may fall victim to secondary infection, exhaustion or malnutrition due to his immobility.

Diagnosis is made by demonstrating the grains extruded from the lesions and further identifying the causative organism by culture. The color of the grains is at times of some diagnostic help. All black grains are due to true fungi and not to the actinomycetes, red grains are produced only by *S. pelletierii*, light-colored grains may be either actinomycetes or true fungi.

More precise identification of the causative organism is afforded by the proper cultural techniques. The aid of a trained mycologist should be utilized to obtain proper culture specimens and to correctly interpret any resulting growth. Fluorescent antibody techniques have been developed to diagnose *A. israelii* infections.

Treatment of mycetoma can be difficult because of fibrosis, abscess formation and bony involvement. Conservative but vigorous medical therapy combined with surgical drainage and débridement should be carried out whenever possible (Fig. 2-17) with amputation only as a last resort.

In general mycetoma due to the actinomycetes responds to therapy much more readily than that due to the true fungi.[1] Mycetoma due to *A. israelii* should be treated with at least 1,000,000 units of penicillin daily with probenecid 1 gm. daily added to decrease renal tubular excretion of penicillin. *N. asteroides* mycetoma should be treated with sulfadiazine in a dose sufficient to yield a blood level of 8 to 12 mg./100 ml. of serum. *N. brasiliensis* mycetoma responds best to the sulfonamides and diaminodiphenylsulfone (D.D.S.).

By and large mycetomas due to the true fungi do not respond to any currently available therapeutic agents, though D.D.S. and the sulfonamides should be tried.

References

1. Zaias, N., Taplin, D., and Rebell, G.: Mycetoma. Arch. Derm., *99*:215, 1969.

VIRAL INFECTIONS

VERRUCAE

Warts are a common nuisance that plague both physician and patient. They are caused by a specific virus (papova virus) that multiplies within the nucleus. Since the average incubation period after experimental inoculation is 4 months, several generations of epidermal cells must undergo inapparent infection.

The virus almost certainly enters the skin directly. One clearly important factor influencing the localization of inoculation of the virus is trauma: nail-biting, occupational trauma, hyperhidrosis or pressure points of the feet. Warts may be transmitted by close contact but the long and variable incubation period and host resistance to infection frequently prevent clear-cut determination of epidemiologic pattern. In some patients, warts are readily autoinoculated. Group pools, gymnasium facilities and locker rooms increase the likelihood of spread of plantar warts. Acuminate warts often, but not always, are spread by sexual contact.

Warts are rather uncommon in infancy and early childhood, reach their peak incidence between age 12 and 16 and then decline in frequency. Rook[1] gives the incidence of the various clinical forms of warts as common warts 70 percent, plantar warts 24 percent, plane warts 3.5 percent, filiform warts 2.0 percent and acuminate warts 0.5 percent. One of the remarkable features of warts is that they may suddenly disappear; the rate of spontaneous regression is probably in the region of 30 percent over a period of 3 to 6 months. The actual mechanism by which warts regress is still not known. Circulating antibodies to the virus in wart-bearing patients have been demonstrated; however, their possible role in immunity and spontaneous regression has not been established.

Common warts most frequently occur on the dorsal surfaces of the hands and on the fingers. They are also often seen on the legs but they may occur on other areas of skin including the face and the dorsal surfaces of the feet and toes. A significant percentage (Rook quotes 65 percent) will disappear spontaneously in 2 years, but many persist indefinitely or require removal for cosmetic reasons or because of obvious autoinoculation.

Plane warts most commonly occur on the face, backs of hands and the shins. The Koebner phenomenon is often noted. Plane verrucae may disappear within a few weeks, or months, or may persist for years and are frequently resistant to therapy. Plane warts usually occur in young children and teen-agers.

The types of warts seen on the feet are the common wart on the dorsum and toes, and the plantar wart with its variant the mosaic wart (Figs. 2-18, 2-19, 2-20). Common warts appear as grey or brown elevated firm papules with horny pitted surfaces. Thrombosed superficial capillaries may produce black or brown specks under the surface. Common warts are frequently multiple and may reach a size of 2

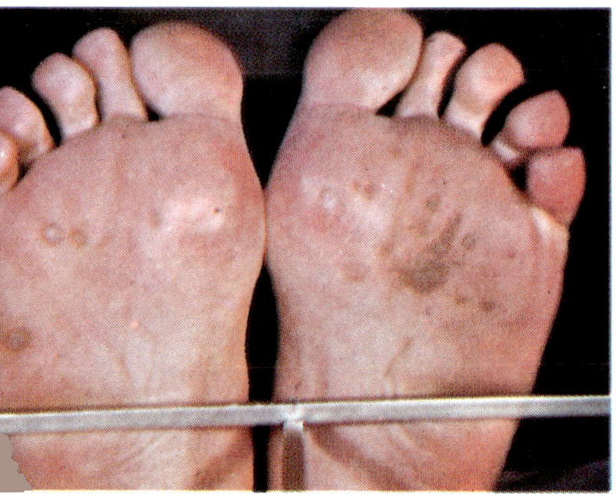

2-18. Typical lesions of plantar verrucae.

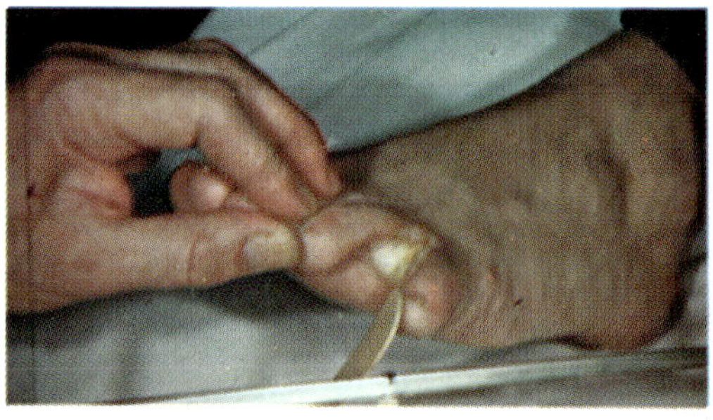

Fig. 2-19. Interdigital verruca. Warts in the web region are frequently misdiagnosed as tinea or maceration.

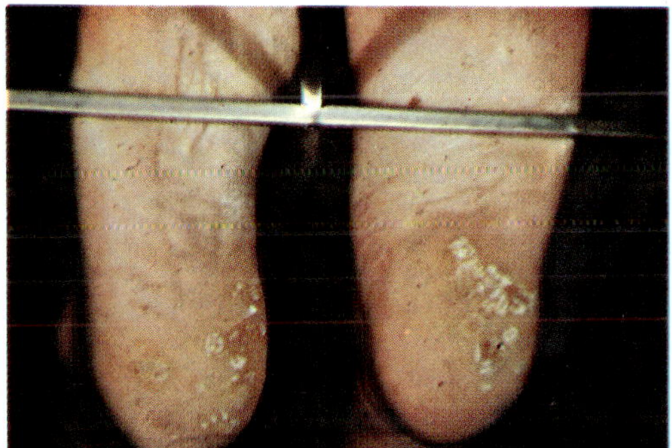

Fig. 2-20. Mosaic verrucae.

centimeters in diameter and one centimeter in height above the skin surface.

Plantar warts occur on the sole, and thereby certain distinctive features are imposed upon them. Besides exposure to the virus, pressure plays an important role, thus accounting for their frequent occurrence most often on points of pressure. It has been noted that women have a higher incidence of plantar warts than do men; high heels could be a factor because the wearing of such heels produces increased pressure on the balls of the feet and big toe. Because they are subjected to frequent heavy pressure from the patient's standing and walking, plantar warts are pushed inward and sideway in the thickened epidermis of the sole and do not grow outward from the skin as is seen with common warts occurring elsewhere. Because of this inward growth and the pressure, plantar warts frequently are tender, occasionally markedly so.

Plantar warts can vary in size from a pinhead to a half-dollar. The majority of patients who have plantar warts have a single lesion. Sometimes a cluster of small satellite warts having a vesicular appearance may develop around a larger wart, so-called mother-daughter warts. When the plantar wart is gently pared, the horny margin is sharply outlined; if the paring is continued, capillary tips perpendicular to the surface are visible. Mosaic warts are often mistaken for calluses, however paring reveals the angular outlines of tightly compressed individual warts that resemble a mosaic. In prepubertal children, plantar warts may disappear in 6 months but in older children and adults they often persist for years.

It is important to distinguish plantar warts from neurovascular corns and callosities. All three lesions occur at pressure points of the sole but the prognosis varies with the diagnosis. Corns and callosities are cutaneous reactions to pressure and relief from pain can be achieved by paring and 40 percent salicylic acid pads under occlusion. Permanent "cure" may require orthopedic devices such as pads or metatarsal bars to remove pressure from the area.

The myriad of therapies for warts attest to the lack of a truly satisfactory form of therapy. The choice will be influenced by the physician's previous experience and preferences, the number of verrucae, the location of the lesions and the age of the patient. Less aggressive techniques should always be used first, especially with children.

For some unknown reason, warts can be cured or "charmed" away by psychotherapy or suggestion. There would appear to be no scientific basis for this effect, and it is impossible to assess the value of the influence of suggestion. Success probably depends on the tendency of warts to spontaneous regression. Nevertheless, if suggestion is applicable to the patient, especially children, it should be considered.

Curettage and light electrodesiccation is the most commonly used therapy for common warts and is generally satisfactory. The desiccation should be gentle to minimize risk of scarring.

Plantar warts are often treated by 40 percent salicylic acid plaster with adhesive tape occlusion or salicylic acid paste with plastic cup occlusion. The softened tissue is then pared by the physician at regular intervals. This mode of therapy is usually painless, does not restrict the patient's activity and there is virtually no risk of scarring. Its only disadvantage is that several weeks to several months therapy may be required. This regimen can be modified by using curettement after one week occlusion with 40 percent salicylic acid. In this method, the skin is prepared with thimerosal and then a local anesthetic such as Xylocaine is injected directly into the wart. The wart is scooped out with a curet; bleeding can be controlled by light desiccation or by application of trichloracetic acid or by pressure with a cotton-tipped applicator. A drop of an antibiotic ointment can then be placed in the cavity which is then covered with a dry dressing. For mosaic warts, we prefer a simple regimen of painting the areas with Castellani's solution in the morning and "sanding" with sandpaper nightly.

Other forms of therapy are formalin soaks, podophyllin with adhesive tape occlusion and the topical application of various acids. Often plantar warts have been surgically excised but this is best reserved for those few cases that do not respond to more conservative forms of therapy, since recurrences are not rare. The procedure is painful and there may be a significant period of postoperative disability and occasionally a painful scar is produced.

Therapy for periungual warts can at times by very difficult. Curettage and electrodesiccation can be used but there is a risk of nail deformity secondary to matrix damage from the procedure. Cantharidin under occlusion, liquid nitrogen freezing and 40 percent salicylic acid under occlusion can also be used. Liquid nitrogen is applied with a cotton-tipped applicator for 10 to 30 seconds with light or moderate pressure. This produces a blister in 1 to 3 days and in about 7 days the wart, along with a piece of the epidermis around it, may be lifted out. At times, the freezing will have to be repeated.

There is no rationale in the use of repeated smallpox vaccinations or any of the present-day agents administered systemically for the treatment of plantar warts. Wart vaccines have been found to be of no specific value. X-ray therapy carries a potential hazard and should not be used. Ultrasound has also been advocated.[2] However experience is limited and the effectiveness of this therapy relative to other forms of treatment cannot be judged.

HERPES SIMPLEX

Primary herpes simplex infection usually is asymptomatic and occurs before the age of 5 years. In a small minority of the population the primary infection manifests itself in one of several forms, usually gingivostomatitis, vulvovaginitis or keratoconjunctivitis. After infection, specific antibodies appear and persist throughout the life of the individual, while a persistent carrier state of the virus in the skin is also believed to occur.

Recurrent episodes of herpes simplex occur in about one percent of the population who possess normal serum antibody levels. Such recurrent lesions usually occur on the face, especially around the mouth, but may develop anywhere on the cutaneous surface, including the feet.

In those persons who experience recurrent herpes simplex infections, one or more of several factors may trigger reactivation of the latent virus. These factors include fever, sunlight, trauma, foods, drugs, menstruation and emotional stress. Many episodes occur without obvious cause.

The clinical appearance of the lesions of herpes simplex on the feet is the same as for other glabrous skin areas; that is, the sudden onset of small grouped clear vesicles on an erythematous base which subsequently dry and form crusts. Sensations of itching and burning accompany the appearance of the lesions. Healing occurs in 7 to 10 days with no resultant scarring. Lesions may occur on the dorsal aspect or sole of the foot. After the lesions appear, they are usually asymptomatic on most areas of the skin but on the distal portions of the extremities they may be associated with fever, pain and lymphangitis. Two particular forms of primary herpes simplex may occur on the foot: inoculation herpes simplex and eczema herpeticum. Direct inoculation of the virus into an abrasion or into normal skin may give rise, after an incubation period of 5 to 7 days, to deep-seated vesicles which are often extremely painful. Regional nodes are often enlarged and the lesion is frequently mistaken for a pyogenic infection. Often it is only after the lesions do not respond to antibacterial therapy that the diagnosis of a primary herpes simplex inoculation infection (herpetic whitlow) is considered. Herpetic whitlows usually occur on the fingers, especially of dentists, physicians, nurses and dental assistants, but rarely on the toes. Eczema herpeticum in which massive crops of vesicles and pustules occur accompanied by severe constitutional symptoms results from herpes simplex infection in patients with preexisting skin disease. The virus enters the skin during the viremic phase but it is felt that autoinoculation is not an important factor. Most cases occur in patients with atopic dermatitis; rarely it may be associated with Darier's disease, pemphigus foliaceus, ichthyosiform erythroderma or other inflammatory dermatoses.

Most lesions of herpes simplex involute without treatment in 8 to 10 days. For the relief of symptoms, simple measures such as drying lotions are preferred during the early vesicular and oozing stage. After drying of the blisters, a lubricating ointment can be used to soften the crusts or an antibiotic ointment to reduce the possibility of secondary bacterial infection.

HERPES ZOSTER

Zoster is caused by the same virus which gives rise to varicella. Varicella usually occurs in childhood and is regarded as the primary infection, while zoster occurs predominantly in adults and is felt to be the reactivation of a latent viral infection. Approximately two-thirds of patients with zoster are over 45 years of age. Patients with lymphomas, particularly Hodgkin's disease, have an increased incidence of zoster and the occurrence of gangrenous or disseminated zoster should raise suspicion of an underlying lymphoma.

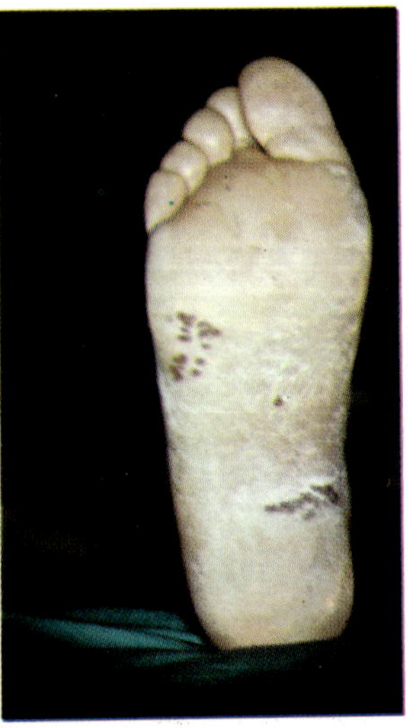

Fig. 2-21. Typical lesions of herpes zoster.

The initial manifestation of zoster is often pain, which may be severe, localized to the area of one or more dorsal roots. After a few days, erythematous papules appear along one or two dermadromes, rapidly becoming vesicular and then pustular. The involvement is usually unilateral except in the rare cases of disseminated zoster. The regional lymph nodes are enlarged and tender. Recovery takes from 2 to 4 weeks but persistent postherpetic pain may be a troublesome or even disabling problem for months, especially among elderly patients. While zoster involves the thoracic, cervical and trigeminal nerves in the great majority of cases, in unusual instances the lesions will involve one leg and extend down onto the dorsum or sole of the foot (Fig. 2-21).

Many initially enthusiastic reports of various therapeutic agents have appeared over the years only to soon fade into oblivion. At the present time the major therapy is symptomatic for relief of pain. The skin lesions are treated much the same as an acute dermatitis: cool, astringent wet compresses applied for 20 minutes 3 or 4 times a day during

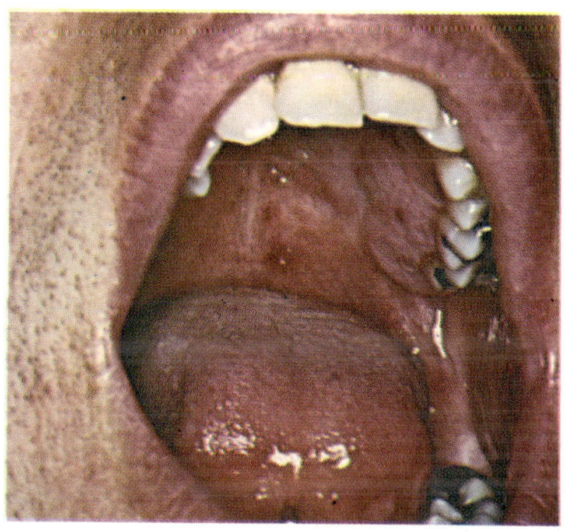

Fig. 2-22. Hand, foot and mouth disease. Mouth lesions. Coxsackie A16 virus isolated.

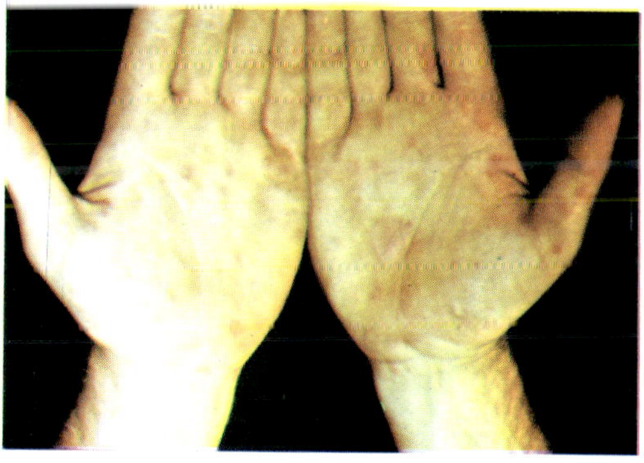

Fig. 2-23. Hand, foot and mouth disease. Hand lesions. Same patient.

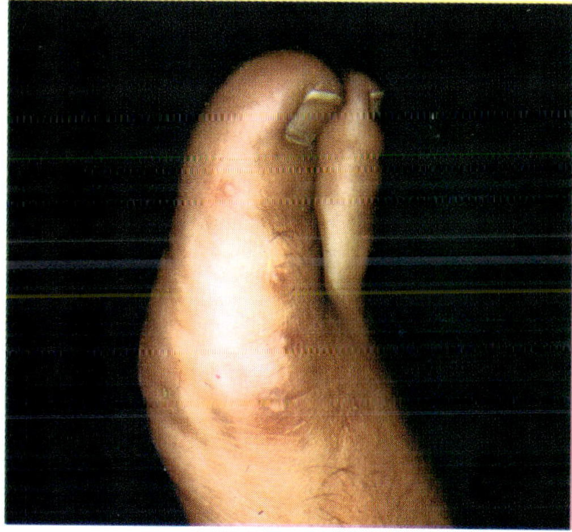

Fig. 2-24. Hand, foot and mouth disease. Foot lesions. Same patient.

the early stages of the eruption. After the lesions have dried, topical steroid creams or antibiotic ointments, when secondary bacterial infection is present, can be helpful.

Some observers feel that systemic steroids administered early in the illness may help to promote healing and reduce the incidence of postherpetic neuralgia; however, the fear of steroids causing dissemination of the viral disease has also been of concern. In a recent double blind study by Eaglstein and associates,[3] patients with early severely painful zoster received either lactose placebos or triamcinolone. The systemic steroids did not cause any worsening of the cutaneous eruption, did not result in quicker healing of the lesions and did not lessen the pain during the first two weeks. However, such therapy did shorten the duration of postherpetic neuralgia in patients over the age of 60.

HAND, FOOT AND MOUTH DISEASE

This disease is usually caused by Coxsackie A16 virus but occasional outbreaks have been reported due to A5 and to other types. A painful stomatitis with irregularly distributed erosions is usually the most prominent feature of the disease. Skin lesions consist of thin walled, light gray vesicles with narrow red areolae and may be present in as few as 25 percent of cases. When they do occur, they usually are located on the dorsal surfaces of the fingers and toes, especially around the nails. Lesions also occur on the palms and soles, in which cases they may be quite tender. Lesions tend to be limited in number, fade in 2 or 3 days and the course of the entire disease is mild and lasts from 4 to 7 days. There is no specific therapy (Figs. 2-22, 2-23, 2-24).

FOOT AND MOUTH DISEASE

Foot and mouth disease due to one of the nonhuman picornaviruses, is an epidemic disease of farm animals which rarely infects man. The disease is usually mild and consists of fever, headache, malaise, burning and vesicles of the oral mucous membranes, tongue and lips. Vesicles also appear on the palms, soles and interdigital skin. The vesicles become ulcers and there may be some pain and edema. There is no specific therapy.

References

1. Rook, A., Wilkinson, D.S., and Ebling, F.J.G.: Textbook of Dermatology. p. 753. Oxford,Blackwell Scientific Publications, 1968.

2. Kent, H.: Warts and ultrasound. Arch. Derm., *100*:79, 1969.

3. Eaglstein, W.H., Katz, R., and Brown, J.A.: The effects of early corticosteroid therapy on the skin eruption and pain of herpes zoster. JAMA, *211*:1681, 1970.

SPIROCHETAL INFECTIONS

Syphilis is caused by infection with the spirochete, *Treponema pallidum*, and is divided into 3 clinical stages — primary, secondary, and late. A complete classification is listed in Table 2-1.* The natural history of syphilis is outlined on Table 2-2.*

PRIMARY SYPHILIS

The chancre of primary syphilis occurs at the site of inoculation and penetration of the skin by the spirochete. Thus, the chancre is usually located on the genitalia; occasionally it may appear on the lips where it may be mistaken for a malignant lesion. However, rarely the chancre may appear elsewhere as on the toe in Figure 2-25. The chancre is an ulcerated or eroded firm papule which is painless. If the lesion is located where regional lymph nodes can be palpated, discrete, rubbery nontender enlarged nodes, the satellite bubo, may be found. The primary chancre will heal from 4 to 6 weeks without therapy, but treatment must be undertaken to prevent the disease from continuing its course.

Serological tests do not become reactive until 1 to 3 weeks after the appearance of the chancre. Thus the tests may be nonreactive in the presence of a syphilitic lesion. Darkfield examination of a chancre will be positive if several attempts are made and if the patient has neither received systemic antibiotics nor applied topical antibiotic ointment to the chancre.

The therapy of choice is a long-acting intramuscular penicillin (Bicillin) given in a single individual dose of 2.4 million units - 1.2 million units into each buttock. In patients who are allergic to penicillin, tetracycline or erythromycin may be given in an oral dose schedule of 2 or 3 grams daily from 10 to 15 days.

SECONDARY SYPHILIS

Approximately 2 months after infection (range: 6 weeks to 6 months), or about 6 weeks after the appearance of the chancre, the lesions of secondary syphilis develop. The eruption is bilaterally symmetrical, rather widespread in distribution, either maculopapular, papular, papulosquamous or, infrequently, pustular. In teen-agers or adults the eruption is never vesicular or bullous. The palms and soles (Fig. 2-26) are commonly involved. Condyloma lata may occur in the anogenital region, around the mouth or occasionally in the toe webs (Fig. 2-27). Lymphadenopathy, hepatosplenomegaly and alopecia may be present. When present they are often accompanied by constitutional symptoms such as fever, malaise and sore throat. All moist lesions of secondary syphilis are highly contagious and darkfield positive. Serologic tests are virtually always reactive at this stage, often in high titer.

*We are indebted to Charles L. Heaton, M.D., Department of Dermatology, University of Pennsylvania for Tables 2-1, 2-2 and 2-3.

CLASSIFICATION

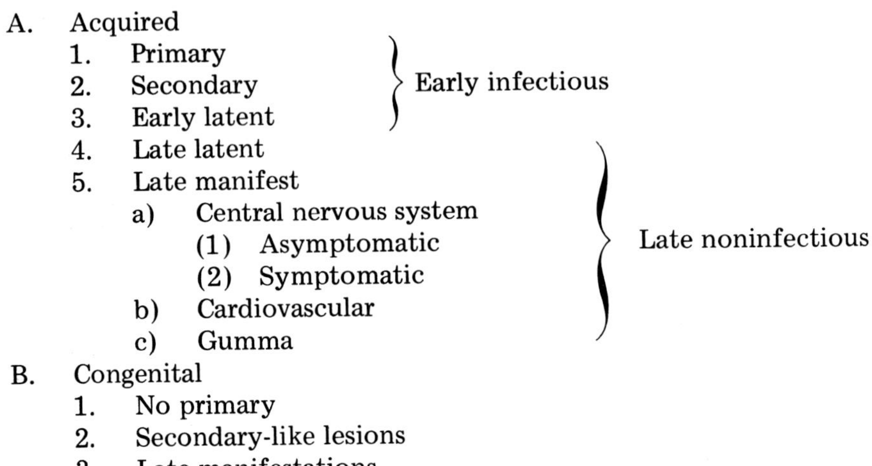

A. Acquired
  1. Primary
  2. Secondary
  3. Early latent
  4. Late latent
  5. Late manifest
     a) Central nervous system
        (1) Asymptomatic
        (2) Symptomatic
     b) Cardiovascular
     c) Gumma

(Primary, Secondary, Early latent: Early infectious)
(Late latent, Late manifest: Late noninfectious)

B. Congenital
  1. No primary
  2. Secondary-like lesions
  3. Late manifestations
  4. Stigmata

Table 2-1

NATURAL HISTORY OF UNTREATED SYPHILIS

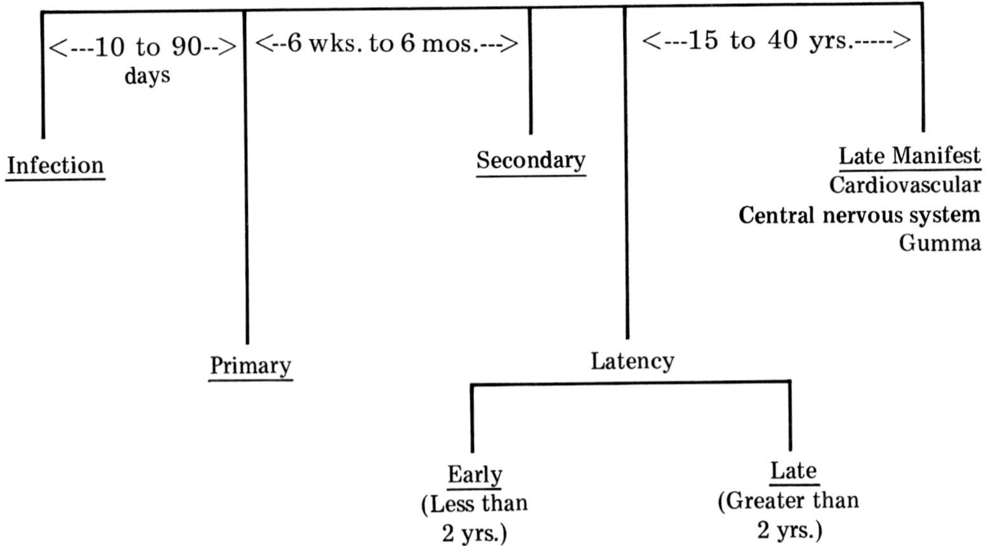

Table 2-2

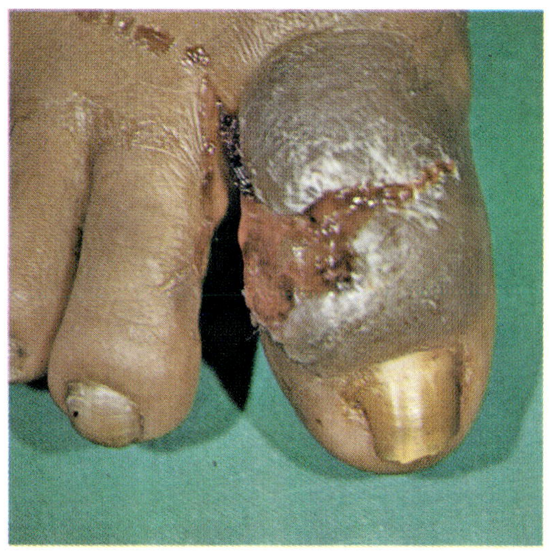

Fig. 2-25. Chancre on toe.

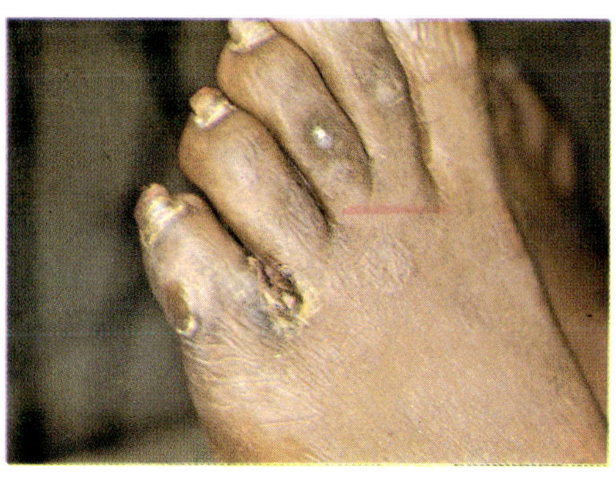

Fig. 2-27. Secondary syphilis. Condyloma lata in the toewebs.

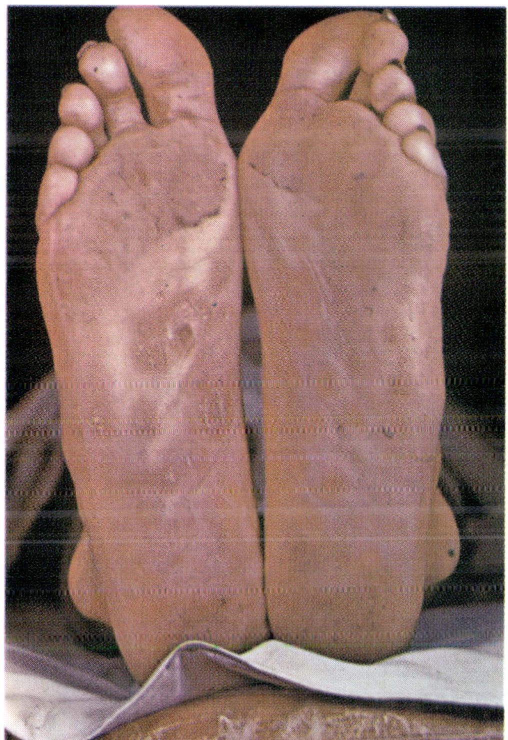

Fig. 2-26. Secondary syphilis. Note characteristic "ham" color of the maculopapular lesions.

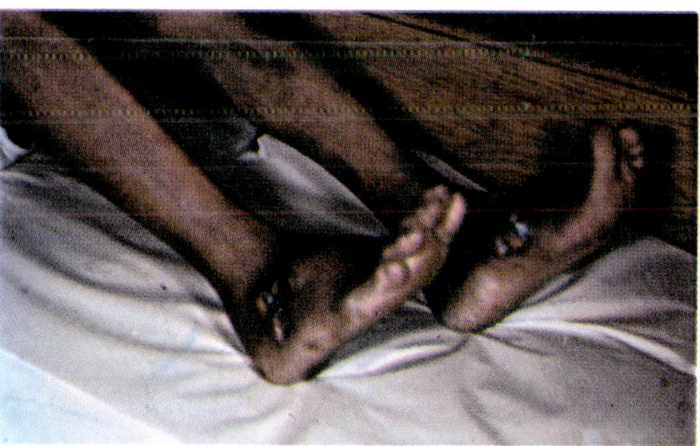

Fig. 2-28. Late syphilis. Multiple gummas. Note the characteristic, indolent, deeply infiltrated and punched-out ulcers.

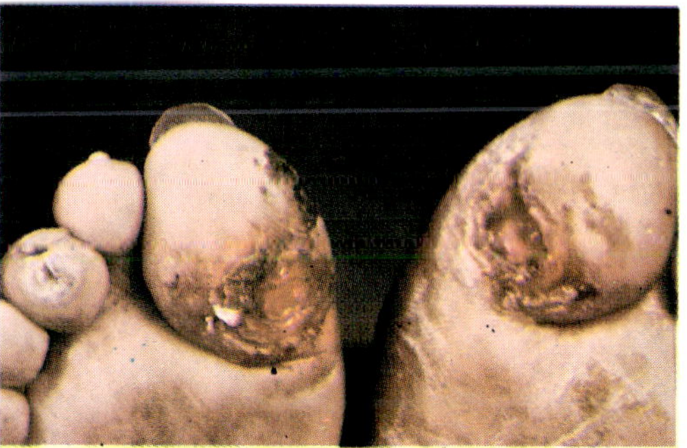

Fig. 2-29. Late syphilis. Mal perforans.

If untreated, the lesions of secondary syphilis will resolve without therapy. Treatment is indicated to prevent progression of the disease and is identical to that for primary syphilis.

LATENT SYPHILIS

In latent syphilis, no lesions, either cutaneous or systemic, are present. The diagnosis depends upon the finding of a positive serologic test for syphilis which is confirmed by one of the specific treponemal tests (TPI or FTA-ABS).

The treatment for early and late latent syphilis is as described for the primary and secondary stages.

LATE MANIFEST SYPHILIS

In contrast to the lesions of primary and secondary syphilis, the manifestations of late syphilis are not infectious but destructive. Imperfect immunity exists in the host who may have cardiovascular or central nervous system involvement or gummatous lesions. Only in gummatous and central nervous system lesions, however, do lesions occur on the lower extremity. In neurosyphilis, there may be hypesthesia or anesthesia of the distal extremities which may lead to trophic ulcers of the feet. Gummata, which represent hypersensitivity reactions to the treponemes, may involve the viscera, skin or bone. Biopsies of chronic granulomatous ulcers of the lower extremity may lead to the diagnosis of a previously unsuspected gumma (Figs. 2-28, 2-29). Gummas show dramatic improvement and healing after the initiation of specific therapy.

In late manifest syphilis the indicated therapy is benzathine penicillin G 2.4 million units intramuscularly weekly for 3 weeks, a total dose of 7.2 million units.

SYPHILIS SEROLOGY (Table 2-3)

It must be stressed that the titer of reactivity of serologic tests for syphilis neither determines the stage of syphilis nor the severity of the patient's infection.

The nontreponemal (reagin or cardiolipin) tests serve as screening tests, and are diagnostic of a treponemal infection only when there is a rapidly rising titer over a 7 to 10 day period. Once the diagnosis of syphilis has been established these tests are most helpful in establishing the adequacy of therapy. Falling titers obtained sequentially at 2 or 3 month intervals indicate adequate therapy.

The specific treponemal tests (TPI and FTA-ABS) are used only to confirm the presence or absence of treponemal antibodies. They thereby confirm a diagnosis of syphilis and rule out a biological false positive reagin test. They cannot be used to determine the activity of syphilis or the adequacy of the patient's therapy.

The reader, who may desire further discussion of serologic tests for syphilis, including sensitivity, specificity and sero-fast states as well as acute and chronic biologic false positive reactions, is referred to standard texts on syphilis.

SEROLOGY

A. Tests
   1. Nontreponemal test - Syn.: Reagin or Cardiolipin Tests
      a) Flocculation - VDRL
      b) Agglutination - RPRC (Rapid Plasma Reagin Card. Test)
      c) Complement-Fixation - Wasserman, Kolmer
   2. Treponemal tests
      a) Whole body virulent viable - TPI
      b) Whole body nonviable - FTS-ABS

B. Interpretation: Consider sensitivity, specificity, significance of titer changes, and sero-fast patients.

C. Biologic False Positive Tests
   1. Acute
   2. Chronic

Table 2-3

MYCOBACTERIAL INFECTIONS

The atypical or anonymous acid-fast mycobacteria, a group of mycobacteria which differ from *Mycobacterium tuberculosis*, *Mycobacterium bovis*, and *Mycobacterium leprae*, are capable of causing a variety of skin lesions in man. Some of the characteristics which differentiate the atypical mycobacteria from *Mycobacterium tuberculosis* are: pretherapy resistance, strong catalase activity, ability to grow at room temperature and inability to produce progressive disease in guinea pigs after subcutaneous inoculation.[1] Mice are more susceptible than guinea pigs to some of the atypical mycobacteria.

The atypical acid-fast mycobacteria have been found in nature in soil, water and excreta. Runyon classified them into four groups.[2] Group I contains the organisms which produce pigment only after exposure to light (photochromogens). Group II contains the organisms which produce pigment regardless of the presence or absence of light (scotochromogens). The pigment produced by Groups I and II is yellow or yellow-orange. Group III is characterized by the absence of pigment formation (nonphotochromogens). Group IV is characterized by the rapid growth of the organism (rapid growers).

M. avium, *M. kansasii*, scotochromogens, *M. intracellulare* (Battey bacillus), and *M. fortuitum* produce primarily pulmonary disease in man. Except with less common disseminated disease, draining sinuses, adenitis, and osteomyelitis these rarely involve the skin of the lower extremity. *M. marinum* and *M. ulcerans* are well-known pathogens which infect the skin. These organisms do not have pulmonary manifestations and therefore were not listed in Runyon's original classification.

In the United States the most frequently recognized lesion is the swimming pool granuloma caused by *M. marinum* (balnei). The lesions develop on traumatized skin and thus occur most frequently on the elbows, knees and dorsal portions of the feet and hands (Fig. 2-30). After a 3 to 4 week incubation period, a small reddish papule(s) appears and slowly increases in size to become a hard purplish nodule(s). This nodule sometimes ulcerates and becomes covered with a scab or greyish exudate or becomes heavily crusted and verrucous in appearance. The

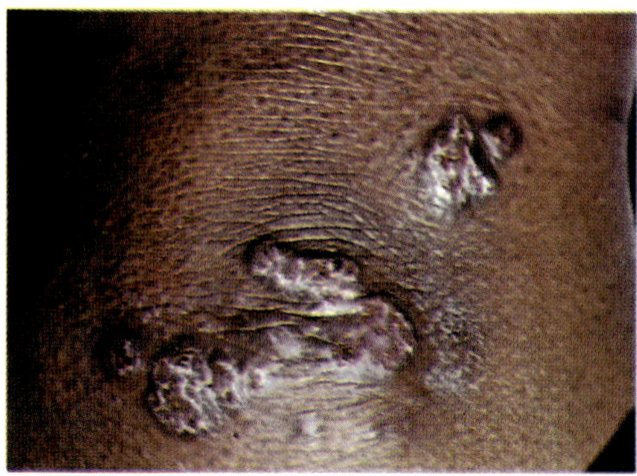

Fig. 2-30. Mycobacterial infection on knee. *M. balnei* cultured.

lesions are usually asymptomatic and are not associated with lymphangitis or regional lymphadenopathy. Healing with scarring occurs after several months in most cases, although there are reports of lesions persisting for 4 to 45 years.[3,4]

In most cases, *M. marinum* has been isolated from crevices and grooves in the cement walls of the pools in which patients had been swimming. Local epidemics have occurred in Sweden and Colorado. Because of the association of this disease with fresh water swimming, the designation "swimming pool granuloma" has been used, although there are cases in which pools have not been the source of the organism.[5,6]

In the tropics, *Mycobacterium ulcerans* infections are highly prevalent in certain localities, and at times are very severe. Most cases occur in children with half of the patients being between 5 and 14 years. Most of the lesions occur on the extremities, about one-half on the lower extremity, usually beginning on the anterior tibial area. Usually the lesions are single and follow minor trauma. In the 3-week period following inoculation, induration develops and extends in diameter and depth. Hyperpigmentation of the overlying skin is usual. A rapidly enlarging area of ulceration ensues, followed by secondary infection, resulting in a granulation area covered with a foul exudate. The ulcer margins are irregular and undermining occurs, extending 10 to 15 cm. with buried pockets of whitish necrotic material. Occasionally, small satellite lesions form with a narrow bridge of undermined skin separating the satellite ulcers from the mother lesion. Regional lymph nodes are rarely enlarged and the patient's general health remains relatively unaffected in spite of the size of the lesion.

Skin tests of a purified protein derivative (P.P.D.) of the organism are usually positive; however, one of the most significant characteristics of the mycobacteria as a group is an antigenic relationship. Cross-reactivity with P.P.D. of other mycobacteria (especially tuberculosis) is quite common[7] and may lead to confusion or a misdiagnosis.[8] Culture characteristics will distinguish between *M. marinum* and other mycobacterial infections of the skin.

As mentioned earlier, most lesions heal without therapy. Antituberculosis therapy has been used, and in some cases "better" healing has been reported,[9] but often the organism is resistant, as shown by sensitivity testing. Except in persistent or severe lesions antituberculosis therapy is not indicated; however, if deemed necessary, sensitivity studies should be carried out. Excision of existing lesions may cause an exacerbation.[10] After establishing a diagnosis, masterful inactivity most often seems the wisest course of treatment.

References

1. Runyon, E.H.: Anonymous mycobacteria in pulmonary disease. M. Clin. N. Amer., *43*:273, 1959.

2. *Ibid.*

3. Sommer, A.F., Williams, R.M., and Mandel, A.D.: Mycobacterium balnei infection. Arch. Derm., *86*:316, 1962.

4. Gould, W.M., McMeekin, D.R., and Bright, R.D.: *Mycobacterium marinum* (*balnei*) infection. Arch. Derm., *97*:159, 1968.

5. Dickey, R.F.: Sporotrichoid mycobacteriosis caused by *M. marinum* (*balnei*) Arch. Derm., *98*:385, 1968.

6. Walker, H.H. *et al.*: Some characteristics of "swimming pool" disease in Hawaii. Hawaii Med. J., *21*:403, 1962.

7. Edwards, L.B., and Krohn, E.F.: Skin sensitivity to antigens made from various acid-fast bacteria. Amer. J. Hyg., *66*:253, 1957

8. Gould, W.M., McKeenin, D.R., and Bright, R.: *Mycobacterium marinum* (balnei) infection. Arch. Derm., *97*:189, 1968.

9. Cott, R.E., Carter, D.M., and Sall, T.: Cutaneous disease caused by atypical mycobacterium: report of two chromagen infections and review of the subject. Arch. Derm., *95*:259, 1967.

10. Mollohan, C.S., and Romer, M.S.: Public health significance of swimming pool granuloma. Amer. J. Public Health, *51*:883, 1961.

PARASITIC INFESTATIONS

The term "creeping eruption" refers to a parasitic larval infestation of the skin which is commonly seen in the southeastern United States, Central America, and in many tropical areas of the world. The disorder is usually due to the migration through the skin of the larvae of the dog and cat hookworm *Ancyclostoma braziliense* and *A. caninum* which produces a characteristic linear inflammatory reaction. The condition is also commonly referred to as "sand worm" or "larva migrans."

Cutaneous larva migrans resulting from exposure to nonhuman strains of *A. braziliense* has a widespread distribution throughout the sandy coastal areas of the United States from southern New Jersey to the Florida Keys of the Atlantic coast and along the entire coastline of the Gulf of Mexico. It extends inland in Texas as far as a line drawn north and south through Dallas and San Antonio. The largest number of cases, however, is found in the vicinity of Jacksonville, Florida. Many other tropical and subtropical coastal regions have reported cases, notably southern Brazil, Uruguay and Argentina. Spain, southern France, South Africa, India, the Philippines and Australia similarly have reported cases.

Exposure results from contact of the human skin with damp sandy soil where the larvae have developed after fecal contamination. Common sites of exposure are found both on bathing beaches and under houses where workers may lie while repairing plumbing fixtures. It may also be picked up by children running barefoot in contaminated areas and may also occur in children's unprotected sandboxes.

The initial sites of the lesions are usually on the uncovered parts of the body, hands, face and feet (Fig. 2-31). Occasionally lesions may be situated on the buttocks or genitals; rarely are the mucous membranes of the nose, mouth and conjunctiva involved.

At each point where the filariform larva of *A. braziliense* invades the skin it produces a red itching papule. In 2 or 3 days the larvae produce a serpiginous tunnel at the dermal-epidermal junction. Manifestations arise from the progression of the larvae and appear as a serpentine linear inflammatory reaction. The larvae precede the inflammation by 1 to 2 cm and may migrate as much as several millimeters to several inches daily. The lesions are moderately to intensely pruritic and secondary impetiginization may occur from scratching. Activity of the larvae may continue for several weeks or months resulting in severe skin involvement. The duration of the untreated disease seems to be related to the environmental temperature. Higher temperature apparently causes increased larval activity with a resultant shorter duration of the disease.

Treatment should begin with a discussion of the obvious: prevention. The wearing of protective clothing when in endemic areas is perhaps the most effective preventive measure. The predisposition of children to run barefoot during the spring and summer explains the high incidence of foot and leg involvement. Other protective measures would include proper covering of children's sandboxes, when not in use, so as to discourage visits by neighborhood animals.

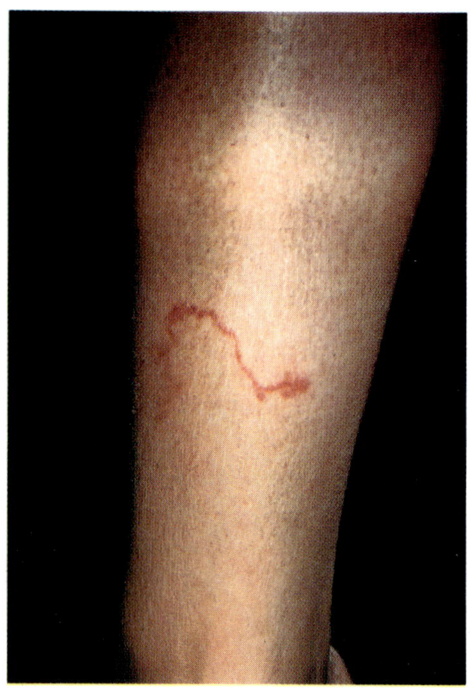

Fig. 2-31. Characteristic lesions of creeping eruption. Acquired by contact with contaminated sand. Topical thiabendazole produced complete healing within 10 days.

Perhaps the most time-honored method of treatment is the application of freezing ethyl chloride spray or the application of dry ice to the "head" of the serpentine lesions. Clinically this is very effective; however, there is little evidence to suggest that this actually kills the larvae. It may be that the inflammatory reaction that follows the freezing aids in the destruction of the organisms.

Hetrazan orally, 2.0 mg. 3 times daily, given after meals for 10 to 20 days has been recommended as a therapeutic measure. More recently thiabendazole has been proven exceptionally effective in the treatment of creeping eruption. It is particularly useful where a patient has infestation which is difficult to manage topically. Side effects are not uncommon with this medication and nausea, vomiting, and dizziness frequently occur. In addition, anorexia and malodorous urine have been reported. The side effects, however, tend to be minimized on a thiabendazole dosage of 25 mg./kg. of body weight for 3 or 4 days.

Pace[1] subsequently reported success in injecting the advancing ends of the burrows with a thiabendazole suspension (100 mg./cc.), using a jet injector. No side effects were noted in his patients and itching was relieved within a few hours after injection. The maximum number of burrows treated in any one patient was about 20. The small amount of drug given to each person (less than 10 mg. per injection) probably accounts for the absence of side effects.

Eyster[2] in 1967 reported success in the treatment of creeping eruption by occlusion of a thiabendazole suspension (Mintezol) and dexamethasone with a polyethylene film. The occlusive dressing was left in place for 3 days. Systemic side effects were absent; however, a few patients developed a symptomless perifollicular eruption which subsided soon after the occlusion was discontinued.

Davis and Israel[3] reported a simple and effective way of using topical thiabendazole. They applied Mintezol sparingly with the fingertips to all lesions 4 times daily. In all patients, pruritus was markedly decreased by the 3rd day of treatment; on the 7th day all lesions were essentially healed. The local and systemic side effects noted in earlier methods of use were not noted, although two patients noted stinging when the medication was applied to denuded areas but it was not severe enough to stop treatment.

Thus, in the common form of creeping eruption, consisting of only a few burrows, simple freezing of the advancing end is a relatively effective simple method of treatment. In more severe infestations, the method of Davis and Israel[4] for topical thiabendazole application appears to be a superior means of management. Only in severe refractory cases should oral thiabendazole be used, since side effects occur rather commonly.

References

1. Pace, B.F.: Creeping eruption treated by jet injection. JAMA, (Letter to the editor), *196*:599, May, 1966.

2. Eyster, W.H.: Local thiabendazole in the treatment of creeping eruption. Arch. Derm., *95*:620, 1967.

3. Davis, C.M., and Israel, R.M.: Treatment of creeping eruption with topical thiabendazole. Arch. Derm., *97*:325, Mar., 1968.

4. *Ibid.*

3

Vascular Disorders

STASIS DERMATITIS

Stasis dermatitis is caused by a disturbance of the normal venous blood flow resulting in an impairment of local tissue physiology and nutrition. It is manifested by pigmentation (hemosiderosis), edema and varicosities (Fig. 3-1). Later, induration (fibrosis) and inflammation occur with or without subsequent ulceration and scarring.

The site of predilection is the lower leg just above the internal malleolus of the ankle, the left more often than the right. It occurs in those middle-aged or older, in women more than men. About one-third of the patients give a definite or suggestive history of deep phlebitis of the limb related to pregnancies, surgery, trauma, or a prolonged illness. In others, varicosities of the primary type or those resulting from increased intra-abdominal pressure (pregnancy, neoplasms, etc.) are present. After a prolonged period of increased pressure in the saphenous system, incompetent perforating veins develop at or near the ankle.

Pigmentation is almost invariably present early. It results from the deposit of hemosiderin following rupture of small venules and presents as a small area of light-brown macules which slowly enlarges as a single patch or by coalescence with other similar areas. Later in the disease, the color is a homogenous darker brown and may cover a very large part of the leg with the lighter brown macules still visible at the periphery. A cyanotic erythema appears, associated with more or less edema which is generally accompanied by pruritus. Scratching may lead to secondary changes, the area becoming thickened and scaly, vesicular or exudative. It is at this time that the injudicious use of topical preparations to combat the pruritus and "infection" presents a major hazard. Sensitization and/or primary irritant reactions are commonly encountered in this situation and are often severe, sometimes with the appearance of distant eczematous patches on the trunk and upper extremities. Once such reaction has occurred, there appears to be a "broadening of the base" so that the patient develops multiple sensitivities.

Edema may not be apparent early, but sooner or later it becomes a prominent feature. It is a basic manifestation of venous insufficiency and leads to a progressive deterioration by mechanically interfering with an already impaired circulation to the local area. Edema from other causes, especially in those with obese legs, is an aggravating factor in many patients. Persons whose occupations require standing for long periods of time, and those who live in a hot and humid environment, are more prone to manifest clinical disease than they would under more favorable circumstances.

Prolonged edema eventually results in fibrosis manifested clinically as an induration or hardening of the tissues. Recurrent episodes of superficial phlebitis add an inflammatory component which, together with the induration, has been referred to as "chronic indurated cellulitis."[1] With each subsequent attack of "cellulitis," fibrosis increases, further impairing local tissue nutrition and slightly retracted whitish sclerotic areas may appear within the hyperpigmented areas. The clinical picture presents as a dermatosclerosis (Fig. 3-2).

Ulceration may result from an episode of "cellulitis," appearing as a superficial, well-demarcated, avascular area. This may heal with scar formation or progress to form a deeper ulcer with soft irregular margins, surrounded by deeply pigmented sclerotic skin. The base is often necrotic and a malodorous discharge is present. Rapid extension with undermining of the edges should arouse suspicion of an infectious process, perhaps of the symbiotic type. In this situation, anaerobic and aerobic cultures, using an adequate inoculum, are almost mandatory. In general, however, infection plays a minor role in stasis ulcer.

A history of slight trauma preceding the appearance of an ulcer is obtained in many patients. The lesion does not heal and there is a slow or rapid extension so that large areas of the lower half of the leg may become involved. Recalcitrant post-traumatic ulcers are more commonly encountered when the disease process has been present for some time and advanced fibrosis and edema are present. It is not unusual to find the new ulcer adjacent to scars of healed lesions.

MANAGEMENT OF STASIS DERMATITIS

The management of stasis dermatitis must be directed to the correction of the basic abnormal physiology of the local tissues and any superimposed complicating factors such as infection or contact dermatitis. The prognosis depends on (1) how early (or late) in the course of the disease the patient is seen; (2) the patient's ability and desire to cooperate; and (3) the skill and knowledge of the therapist.

The prevention of iliofemoral thrombophlebitis would appreciably reduce the incidence of stasis dermatitis. This effort rightly falls into the domain of the surgeon, obstetrician, and internist who are making encouraging progress toward this end. Early ambulation especially has contributed to a lower incidence and prompt attention to other predisposing factors when edema first appears, often only detectable in the evening, is of the utmost importance. This may require the development of new habits or even a change in occupation, if necessary, to eliminate long periods of standing without relief. Periods of lying down or sitting with the feet elevated to the level of the heart are recommended and can be readily accomplished with the aid for instance of the newer reclining chairs. The patient must understand that the normal sitting position, with the feet on the floor or low ottoman, provides no advantage over standing.

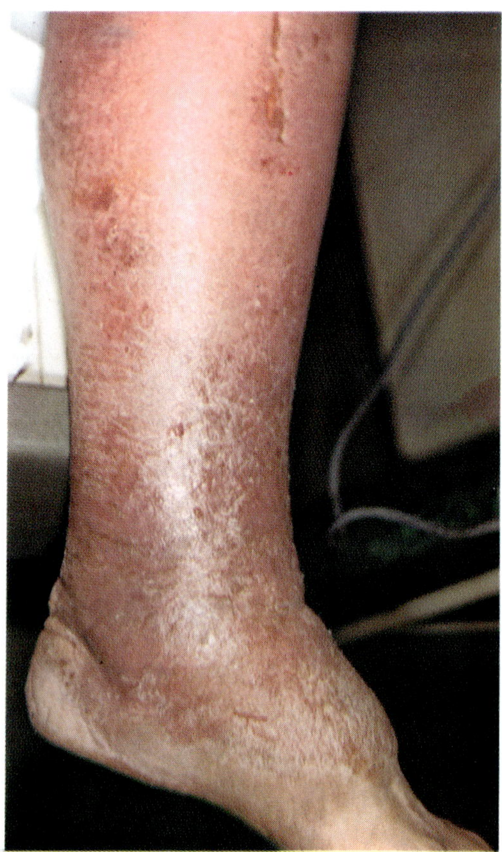
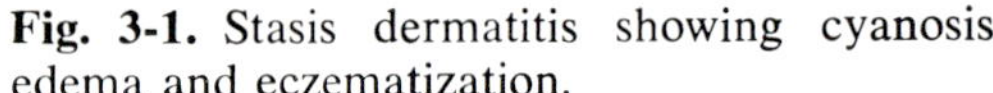

Fig. 3-1. Stasis dermatitis showing cyanosis, edema and eczematization.

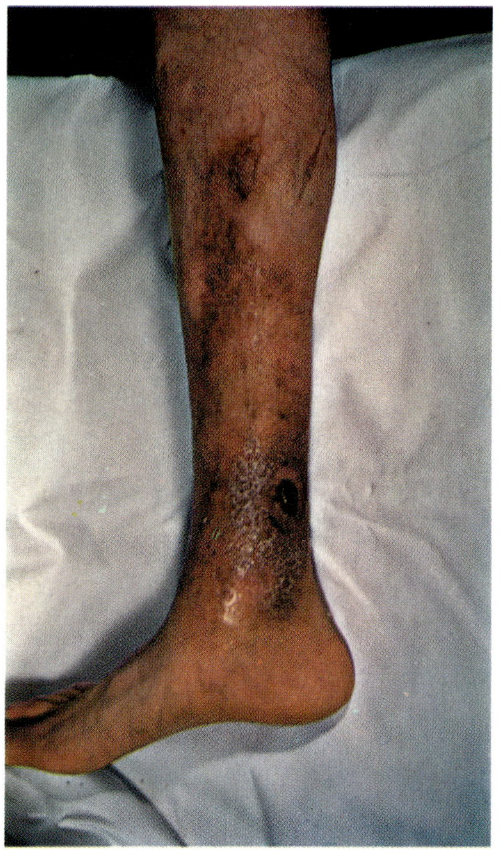

Fig. 3-2. Stasis dermatitis. Chronic stage is characterized by fibrosis and dermatosclerosis.

When the patient presents with well-established stasis dermatitis, whether recent or of long duration, with or without ulceration, the reduction of edema and its subsequent prevention is the first order of importance. When swelling is severe, it may be necessary to put the patient on bed rest, with the foot of the bed elevated 6 to 8 inches, until all swelling has subsided. This period should be as short as possible, preferably no longer than 2 or 3 days, since prolonged inactivity may favor thrombophlebitic processes. The period of bed rest provides an excellent opportunity to correct local infection and/or any eczematous dermatitis.

Local treatment will depend upon the stage of eczematization.

For the acute weeping stage:

Moist cool compresses applied every 3 to 4 hours for 20 minutes. The following solutions are suitable in most cases: (1) isotonic saline solution (0.9 percent); (2) Burow's solution (1:32 or 1:16). Impervious dressings should not be applied because they prevent evaporation, and maceration of the skin may result. If indicated, Burow's paste may be applied between compresses. Antibiotic therapy, local or systemic, is only rarely indicated and its use must be decided on for the individual patient. Avoid aggressive treatment.

For the subacute or chronic stages:

Corticosteroid creams may be alternated with wet dressings and later, with improvement, used alone. Following involution of the stasis dermatitis, the integrity of skin texture can be maintained by a hydration regimen (see under asteatotic eczema).

If secondary sensitization or irritant reactions develop, it is advisable to discontinue all topical applications except simple compresses. Systemic corticosteroid therapy may be indicated in selected cases.

After the edema has subsided, adequate compressive support of the leg is applied just before getting out of bed. There are many methods of supportive therapy, each with its own advocate and, indeed, used successfully by those well versed in their proper application. In the presence of an exudative and inflammatory dermatitis, in which continuation of local therapy is desirable on an ambulatory basis, the use of the elastic bandage is preferred. This can be adjusted with each application whether a paste or other dressing is used under it. The new ACE bandage with Spandex appears to be an improvement over the previous types. In hot weather the use of the all-cotton type may be better tolerated. The bandage must be applied smoothly without any wrinkles, beginning at the base of the toes and extending to the knees, overlapping half a width each turn. Inclusion of the lower part of the thigh has been recommended by some but, from a practical point of view, this is difficult to do well and is rarely accomplished. Their proper application is the keystone to the success of this treatment, but most patients readily accomplish this feat. These bandages must be washed frequently, so that several are required. It is important to replace bandages when they begin to lose their elasticity.

Under certain circumstances the use of an elastic bandage may be inadvisable, (e.g., when the patient lacks the ability to master its application or will not cooperate fully). In such situations the use of an Unna Paste Gelatin Boot is an excellent substitute. Its proper application by the physician insures a safe, adequate support and provides for periodic follow up inspection, preferably weekly, although the initial boot or two may have to be replaced sooner. Active infection must be cleared before starting the therapy. Prepared gelatin bandages (Dome-Paste, Gelocast, etc.) are available and greatly simplify the application of a boot. They should be applied directly to the skin without underlying dressings, even though there still may be active exudation present. Enough layers of the bandage must be used to insure sufficient thickness for adequate support and to prevent creases. To those trained in their proper application, a plaster of paris cast is also effective. This approach has recently been advocated by Menendez[2] who allows them to remain in place for one month, and as long as two months if necessary.

After healing of the dermatitis (and ulcer) has been accomplished, a properly fitted elastic stocking can be prescribed. To be effective, this requires a customized fitting which is possible in most cities. Pressure-gradient support (Jobst) is more satisfactory and effective when prolonged use is necessary. The use of stock elastic stockings is rarely satisfactory and cannot be recommended.

In selected patients, surgical intervention by a knowledgeable surgeon can be of immeasurable help, but the results will depend on the aforementioned factors.

References

1. Ormsby, O.S., and Montgomery, H.: Diseases of the Skin. ed. 8. Philadelphia, Lea & Febiger, 1954.

2. Menendez, C.V.: Ulcers of the Leg. Springfield, (Ill.), Charles C Thomas, 1967.

HUNTING REACTION

In recent years several middle-aged patients have been seen with a clinical syndrome of erythematous, swollen, tender toes, associated with a sensation of burning, stinging, or pain, without preliminary blanching or subsequent cyanosis. The clinical features were either absent or markedly reduced on arising, progressed during the day, and reached maximum intensity in the late afternoon and evening. A marked increase in symptoms was experienced upon exposure of the feet to a cold environment, particularly when going out-of-doors in winter. Occasionally, partial relief was noted from wearing slippers. The symptoms markedly regressed or completely disappeared during the spring and summer with the onset of warm weather and the wearing of sandals or loose shoes. The patient showed no evidence of peripheral vascular disease, venous stasis, connective tissue diseases, dysproteinemias, or neurologic disorders. Pernio and acrocyanosis are not consistent with the clinical picture presented by these patients, since these syndromes are manifested by definite cyanosis and often exhibit associated hyperhidrosis. In addition, infiltrated macules and papules which may be followed by vesicles, and bullae and ulceration are observed in pernio. Some clinicians state that acrocyanosis is not painful or associated with burning or stinging sensations, though others do describe pain as a part of the syndrome.

The first report of this phenomenon was published by Sir Thomas Lewis in his classic paper, "Observations Upon the Reactions of the Vessels of the Human Skin to Cold."[1] It was Lewis who discovered and first described the "hunting phenomenon," which will be postulated as the factor underlying the syndrome in these patients.

Case Report. A 40-year-old woman came to see us in December 1964, and was seen subsequently during the winter months of 1965 and 1966 because of pain in her toes. Approximately 10 years earlier she had first noted bilateral swelling, redness, and burning pain in the 5th toes on exposure to cold in the winter. Within a few years the same symptoms and signs occurred in her great toes and shortly thereafter all her toes became involved. She had noted that exposure to cold weather or pressure from tight boots increased her symptoms. An uncertain history of her feet being severely chilled as a child was obtained, but no definite history of frostbite or other cold injury could be elicited. She had been in good health and the remainder of her past history was unremarkable. On examination, there was slight edema and congestion in the distal portions of the toes (Fig. 3-3). Peripheral pulses were normal. No ulcerations or trophic changes were seen. Physical examination, including the fingers and hands, revealed no other abnormalities.

The following analyses gave normal values: hemoglobin, white blood count, differential, urinalysis, FBS, two-hour postprandial blood sugar, blood urea nitrogen, serum uric acid, serologic test for syphilis, cholesterol, sedimentation rate, serum albumin and globulin including protein electrophoresis, glucose tolerance test, protein-bound iodine, lupus erythematosus preparations on three occasions, stools for occult blood,

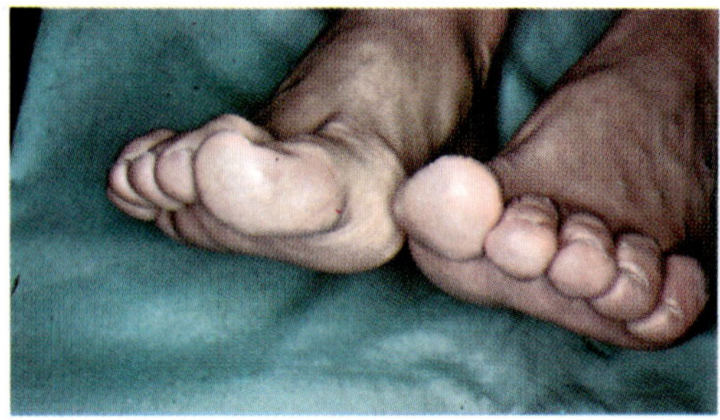

Fig. 3-3. Hunting reaction. Slight edema and congestion of distal portion of toes.

cold agglutinins, cryoglobulins, chest x-ray, and electrocardiogram. A vasodilatation test was normal. Oscillometry revealed oscillations which were perhaps somewhat smaller than normal but not definitely abnormal.

Attempts were made to reproduce the signs and symptoms by blowing cold air on her feet for 30 minutes, immersing the feet in ice water for 15 minutes, and by soaking the feet in 40° to 50° F. water 4 times a day for 2 days. These attempts were unsuccessful. A cardiovascular consultant was uncertain about the diagnosis and believed that the condition was caused by a neurovascular rather than an anatomic abnormality. The patient was discharged and subsequently has continued to experience recurrent symptoms in her toes during cold weather.

In general, the purpose of the circulatory system is to supply oxygen and nutrients to every cell of the organism and to remove the toxic waste products of cellular metabolism. Since different tissues have vastly different requirements under a wide range of diverse conditions, the circulation must be subject to numerous controls. This local regulation of peripheral blood flow is achieved through the coordinated effects of several distinct systems, such as the sympathetic nervous system, local chemical substances in the tissues, and factors acting on intrinsic properties of the vessels themselves.

Zweifach[2] has presented a schematic concept of the pattern of cutaneous vessels (Fig. 3-4). From terminal arterioles emerge metarterioles, or "preferential" thoroughfare channels, which are vessels surrounded by one layer of smooth muscle. The most direct channels from arterial to venous circulation give off side branches called precapillary sphincters, which control the flow of blood into the capillaries proper. The capillaries, consisting only of an endothelial tube, may anastomose and then join the collecting venules. Thus, capillary blood flow can be regulated by the contraction and dilatation of the venules and the precapillary sphincters. Contraction of the precapillary sphincters alone shunts the blood through a preferential channel, bypassing the various lateral capillary networks. Contraction of the metarteriole could shunt the blood arteriovenous anastomoses directly to muscular venules. The venules of the skin, in contrast to those of other tissues, have the ability to contract and dilate.[3]

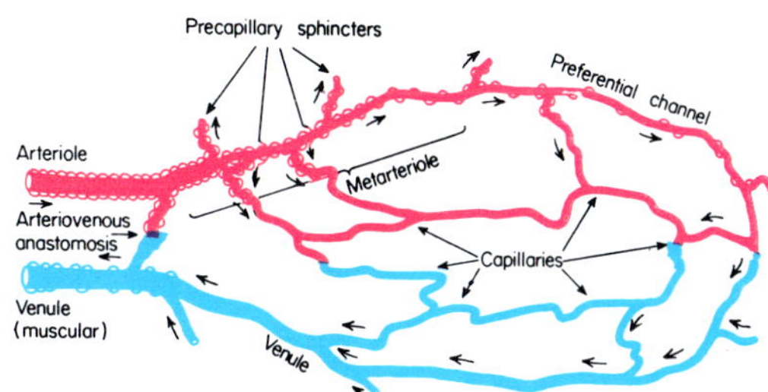

Fig. 3-4. Hunting reaction. Zweifach's concept of the basic structural pattern of the terminals of cutaneous vessels. The white humps on the walls of the vessels indicate muscle fibers.

Compared with other tissues of the body, the cells of the skin require a very low minimum blood flow to maintain their viability — roughly estimated as 0.8 cc./min./100 cc. of skin tissue.[4] The blood flow of the digits varies from a minimum of 0.5 to 1.0 cc./min./100 cc. of tissue in full vasoconstriction to a maximum of 90 cc./min./100 cc. of tissue in full vasodilation. By heat acclimatization this flow can be further increased to 122 cc./min./100 cc. of tissue.[5] Thus, the blood flow through the skin can increase by a factor of 100 to 200. Short variations in blood flow can amount to as much as 20 percent, though they are much less during periods of extreme vasoconstriction or dilatation. Neither this tremendous range nor fluctuation of blood flow is necessary for the maintenance of the cellular metabolic needs of the skin. The minimal flow would be sufficient for normal cellular needs; the maximal flow far exceeds the maximal requirements of the cells. The primary function of vascular control in the skin is, therefore, in the service of the organism as a whole and not of the skin itself. This primary function is temperature regulation. The numerous arteriovenous anastomoses in the skin of the acral areas serve an important role in the ability of the cutaneous vasculature to dissipate or conserve heat as dictated by the needs of the organism.[6] These anastomoses open under the influence of cold and greatly increase the blood flow by shunting blood directly from the arterial to the venous vessels, thereby bypassing the resistance of the capillary bed.

Although the major function of the cutaneous circulation, temperature regulation, serves the organism as a whole, mechanisms for fulfilling local needs are provided as a protective measure against skin damage. One of these mechanisms is the "hunting reaction" of Lewis, a cold-induced paradoxical cyclic vasodilation.

In 1930, Sir Thomas Lewis[7] described an unusual reaction of the cutaneous blood vessels upon cold exposure which resulted in a paradoxical cold-induced cyclic vasodilatation: when a finger is immersed in water sufficiently cold to provide an adequate stimulus (0° to 7°C.), intense vasoconstriction will occur and the skin temperature will drop to within 2 to 4 degrees of the water temperature. However, within 5 to 10 minutes the skin temperature of the digit will begin to rise due to vasodilatation of the cutaneous vessels.

However, with continued immersion, the temperature drops again in several minutes and may reach the original low point, although usually it does not. "It is frequent for the temperature reaction to be repeated over and over again during immersion; this slow 'hunting' of temperature is never quite rhythmic and the rise is irregular in time and form."[8]

Accompanying the temperature changes of the hunting reaction there are also changes in color and subjective symptoms. Soon after immersion the digits begin to ache; the pain increases in severity until the temperature stops falling, and then disappears at or near the turning point of the temperature. As the temperature rises, the fingers or toes become more comfortable and warmer and then begin to burn and throb as the skin becomes erythematous. (Similar sensations and reddening occur in hands which have recently handled snow or been in ice water.) Over the next 4 to 6 minutes the erythema fades with relief of unusual sensations and the digit appears normal well before the temperature begins to return to normal.

The original findings of Sir Thomas Lewis have been confirmed by numerous investigators and thus the existence of the paradoxical cold-induced vasodilatation, commonly called the hunting reaction, is now rather generally accepted. Most, though not all, physicians and physiologists interested in the field of cold injury believe that this vascular response to cold is a protective physiologic mechanism. As this phenomenon acts for local protection at some presumed disadvantage to the organism, Burton[9] considers it a physiologic accident rather than a protective adaptation.

The mechanism by which cold-induced cyclic vasodilatation is produced is not well understood. Lewis originally postulated that the phenomenon was due to both an axon reflex in sensory nerves and to a central nervous system mechanism. Subsequent studies[10,11] showed that the hunting reaction could occur without a nerve supply although the presence of nerves modified the reaction. The vasodilatation occurs asynchronously in the various fingers or toes suggesting that central neural or humoral control is not a factor.[12,13,14,15] However, some investigators[16,17] have reported a significant effect on the hunting reaction from emotional stress, eating, exercise or season of the year. Several chemical substances, including histamine, acetylcholine[18] and bradykinin,[19,20] have been postulated as significant mediators but the evidence has not been convincing.

In a relatively recent article, Folkow *et al.*[21] pointed out that on the basis of the available evidence, the reaction is very complex, involving a number of factors which sometimes are additive in their effects and sometimes counteract each other. Furthermore, the relative importance of each factor can vary according to the particular circumstances; some actually may be absent without changing the trend of the net response.

There seems little doubt that the hunting reaction serves a useful physiologic purpose in protecting the peripheral parts of the body and their integument against damage from exposure to cold. Laboratory studies have shown that when rabbits which are acclimatized in the cold are placed in a cold room (-45° C.) the temperature of their ears remains normal, while nonacclimatized rabbits develop frostbitten ears even though their colonic temperatures are the same as those of the acclimatized rabbits.[22] In experimental cold exposure of the fingers,[23] several features were noted: in acclimatized persons, spontaneous rewarming occurred earlier, proceeded at a more rapid rate, higher and more labile final temperature levels were obtained, faster cooling initially occurred, the cycling time shortened, and pain diminished or disappeared on chronic cold exposure. The inference drawn was that the blood flow was elevated in chronically cold, exposed fingers. The ability of the blood vessels to constrict maximally was not destroyed on chronic cold exposure, but rather was reset at a different level of activity. Similar findings have been noted in the toes. In people indigenous to cold regions, the hunting reaction is very marked. There is increased blood flow in the digits, a more rapid cycling time, more rapid rewarming of the cooled digits, and the extremities are maintained at a warmer temperature in the cold. Thus, these people suffer much less discomfort from the cold without any real danger to the total heat economy of the body.

It would not seem surprising that in an occasional person, a normal protective physiologic mechanism might become excessively active or hypersensitive to the point where the person would experience, in exaggerated form, the sensations that accompany the hunting reaction. Thereby he would develop unpleasant symptoms of pain and throbbing along with color changes of the digits upon slight cold exposure or pressure from shoes.

References

1. Lewis, T.: Observations upon the reactions of the vessels of the human skin to cold. Heart, *15*:177, 1929-31.

2. Zweifach, B.W.: Structural aspects and hemodynamics of microcirculation in the skin. *In* Rothman, S. (ed.): The Human Integument, Washington, DC: American Association for the Advancement of Science, No. 54, pp 67-76, 1959.

3. *Ibid.*

4. Burton, A.C.: Physiology of cutaneous circulation, thermoregulatory functions. *In* Rothman, S. (ed.): The Human Integument, Washington, DC: American Association for the Advancement of Science, No. 54, pp 77-88, 1959.

5. *Ibid.*

6. Rothman, S., and Lorincz, A.L.: Defense mechanisms of the skin. Ann. Rev. Med., *14*:215, 1963.

7. Lewis, T.: Observations upon the reactions of the vessels of the human skin to cold. Heart, *15*:177, 1929-31.

8. *Ibid.*

9. Burton, A.C., and Eagan, C.J.: The Operation of Arterio-venous Anastomoses and the Hunting Reaction of Lewis, in the Proceedings of the International Physiology Congress, Brussels, p 150, 1956.

10. Duff, F., *et al.*: The response to vasodilator substances of the blood vessels in fingers immersed in cold water. J. Physiol., *121*:46, July, 1953.

11. Edholm, O.G., in discussion, Schumacker, H.B., Jr.: Animal studies. *In* Ferrer, M.I. (ed.): Cold Injury: Transactions of the First Conference. pp 17-57. New York, Josiah Macy, Jr., Foundation, 1951.

12. Duff, F., *et al.*: The response to vasodilator substances of the blood vessels in fingers immersed in cold water. J. Physiol., *121*:46, July, 1953.

13. Edholm, O.G., in discussion, Shumacker, H.B., Jr.: Animal studies. *In* Ferrer, M.I. (ed.): Cold Injury: Transactions of the First Conference. pp 17-57. New York, Josiah Macy, Jr., Foundation, 1951.

14. Adams, T., and Smith, R.E.: Effect of chronic local cold exposure on finger temperature responses. J. Appl. Physiol., *17*:317, Mar., 1962.

15. Blair, J.R., in discussion, Shumacker, H.B., Jr.: Animal Studies. *In* Ferrer, M.I. (ed.): Cold Injury: Transactions of the First Conference, pp 17-57. New York, Josiah Macy, Jr. Foundation, 1951.

16. Meehan, J.P.: Avenues of heat loss and peripheral circulation. *In* Ferrer, M.I. (ed.): Cold Injury: Transactions of the Fifth Conference. pp 291-320. New York, Josiah Macy, Jr. Foundation, 1957.

17. Yoshimura, H., and Iida, T.: Studies on the reactivity of skin vessels to extreme cold: Part I. A point test on the resistance against frost bite, Jap. J. Physiol., *1*:147, Aug., 1950-1951.

18. Duff, F., *et al.*: The response to vasodilator substances of the blood vessels in fingers immersed in cold water. J. Physiol., *121*:46, July, 1953.

19. Fox, R.H., and Hilton, S.M.: Bradykinin formation in human skin as a factor in heat vasodilatation. J. Physiol., *142*:219, July, 1958.

20. Fox, R.H., Goldsmith, R., and Kidd, D.J.: Cutaneous vasomotor control in the human head, neck and upper chest. J. Physiol., *161*:298, May, 1962.

21. Folkow, B., *et al.*: Studies on the reactions of the cutaneous vessels to cold exposure. Acta Physiol. Scand., *58*:342, Aug., 1963.

22. Blair, J.R., in discussion, Shumacker, H.B., Jr.: Animal studies. *In* Ferrer, M.I. (ed.): Cold Injury: Transactions of the First Conference. pp 17-57. New York, Josiah Macy, Jr., Foundation, 1951.

23. Adams, T., and Smith, R.E.: Effect of chronic local cold exposure on finger temperature responses. J. Appl. Physiol., *17*:317, Mar., 1962.

VASCULITIDES (Necrotizing)

One outstanding feature of the disorders included under the term "vasculitis" is the confusion engendered by the proliferation of synonyms, eponyms and pseudoentities ascribed to clinical variations.

In 1866, Kussmaul and Maier described a disease of unknown etiology and called it "periarteritis nodosa." In 1925, Gruber suggested that periarteritis nodosa might represent a systemic hyperallergic reaction to various infections and toxic agents to which the blood vessel walls had been exposed previously. In 1942, Rich noted necrotizing vascular lesions which he called "periarteritis nodosa" in serum sickness (thereby confirming the earlier observations of Clark and Kaplan), and in cases of sulfonamide hypersensitivity; in the following year Rich and Gregory produced necrotizing angiitis in rabbits by injecting large amounts of horse serum intravenously. In subsequent years, many cases of angiitis were classed as periarteritis nodosa, though often their clinical features did not resemble the original description of that disease.

In 1952, Zeek reviewed the problem of periarteritis nodosa and stated that much confusion had been created by including under that term a conglomerate of syndromes, many of which were probably separate entities. She suggested the term "necrotizing angiitis" and advocated its use because no particular etiology was implied and the term was applicable to any type or size blood vessel anywhere in the body.[1] Under this generic term, she included five diseases: periarteritis nodosa, hypersensitivity angiitis, rheumatic arteritis, allergic granulomatous arteritis, and temporal arteritis.

Another group of diseases was characterized by granulomatous vasculitis including Wegener's granulomatosis, lethal midline granuloma, and allergic granulomatosis; the relation of these states to each other and to the necrotizing angiitides was, and still is, not clear.

Other forms of necrotizing vasculitis have been reported under the names arteriolitis allergica of Ruiter, dermatitis nodularis necrotica, nodular dermal allergide, anaphylactoid purpura, acute parapsoriasis, allergic microbid, erythema elevatum diutinum, extracellular cholesterosis, and pyoderma gangrenosum.

These numerous syndromes were believed related to each other by the histologic common denominator of necrotizing angiitis. Microscopic examination reveals a marked inflammatory infiltrate in and around the vessel walls, consisting predominantly of polymorphonuclear leukocytes, including numerous eosinophils. The leukocytes become fragmented, and nuclear debris is seen (leukocytoclasis). Extravasation of erythrocytes is an important feature. Necrosis takes place in the wall of the blood vessels, and hyalinization in and around the vessels is seen. Often a wide band of homogenization of connective tissue appears around the involved blood vessels. With the passage of time, a histiocytic response to the amorphous necrotic material may occur and lead to the formation of granulomas.

However, recently Copeman and Ryan[2] discussed some of the misconceptions confusing the classification and understanding of these disorders. They point out that the varied manifestations of the syndromes grouped as cutaneous vasculitis or angiitis are not discrete disease entities and are not confined to the skin but rather are often manifestations of one of several systemic disorders, such as malignancies or collagen diseases. Further attempts at classifying these syndromes clinically or histologically have been unsatisfactory, since no individual clinical or histologic feature is a unique or even a consistent part of any single syndrome. The vasculitis seen in the skin may present as a variety of reaction patterns in one person at the same time. Thus, lesions ranging from urticaria to purpura to bullae may be noted, further stressing the difficulties of attempting rigid clinical classification. Also, the site of the pathology may include capillaries, venules and arteries alone or in any combination.

Thus the diverse manifestations of vasculitis must depend on a number of variables including the type and intensity of the reaction in the vascular wall, the location of the vessel, the duration of the disease, the location and distribution of lesions, the persistence of etiologic agents in the body, and the degree to which the reaction may have been modified by therapy with corticosteroids.[3] Through various combinations of these variables, differing clinical syndromes may result, though the basic pathogenic mechanism may be similar in all cases.

The clinical features of the numerous necrotizing angiitides are extremely protean. Excellent reviews of the diverse manifestations of the various syndromes are by Winkelmann and Ditto,[4] O'Duffy and coworkers,[5] Alarcon-Segovia and Brown,[6] Winkelmann,[7] McCarthy,[8] and, more recently, by Champion and Wilkinson[9] and Borrie and Stansfeld.[10] Copeman and Ryan[11] have presented an interesting classification and discussion of cutaneous vasculitis based on the factors which initiate and then enhance fibrin and platelet deposition and the subsequent pathologic changes resulting from such deposition.

In the remainder of this discussion we shall confine our descriptions to lesions of legs.

The cutaneous lesions include papules, plaques, nodules, petechiae, ecchymoses, vesicles, bullae, urticaria, and necrotic ulcerations. Frequently the evolution of lesions is from petechiae or papules to vesicles and bullae or to nodules and plaques with ulceration. Hemorrhage into the skin is always present.

The lesions are microinfarcts of the skin from vascular occlusion and are most common on the legs, particularly the lower legs, though they may be seen on any part of the body. The skin lesions are usually, but not invariably, bilateral and symmetrical. The onset is often abrupt, the lesions tend to occur in crops, and the episodes may recur. Occasionally, patients notice some sensation in the involved area variously described as itching, burning or stinging. At times pain is mentioned, usually associated with ulceration. Edema, muscular aching, and cramping and arthralgias are also often described.

Over the years numerous etiologies for necrotizing angiitis have been postulated, remained temporarily in vogue, and then passed by the wayside. A significant number of patients have an unmistakable drug reaction (e.g., penicillin, sulfonamides, other antibiotics, phenylbutazone, propylthiouracil) at the time of onset of their vasculitis. Recently necrotizing angiitis has been reported associated with drug abuse.[12] The exact etiology in these cases is not clear, however, methamphetamine appears to be a common denominator. Other patients have an antecedent infection whose onset is closely related to the appearance of the vasculitis. Winkelmann has reported cases of vasculitis from exposure to chlordane, lindane, and 2,4-D, after injection of bacterial desensitization products for chronic sinusitis and following the injection of trypsin.[13]

An interesting hypothesis is that some cases of cutaneous vasculitis represent a Shwartzman reaction. The histologic findings in the Shwartzman reaction are multiple fibrin thrombi in small blood vessels.[14] These changes occur in sites previously prepared by prior exposure to certain toxic or infectious substances. This type of mechanism was postulated by Gruber in 1925. Binkley[15] also invoked this etiologic hypothesis in cases of dermatitis nodularis necrotica. Pyoderma gangrenosum and other cutaneous vasculitides associated with ulcerative colitis have been considered by some to be forms of the Shwartzman phenomenon initiated by unknown products absorbed from the diseased colon which act as antigens.[16,17] Copeman and Ryan[18] have discussed the possible roles of antigen-antibody complexes, bacterial endotoxin and trauma on the initiation of fibrin and platelet deposition and the role of impaired fibrinolysis, abnormal plasma globulins, increased red cell viscosity, increased blood viscosity and stasis, gravity and external pressure on enhancement of fibrin and platelet deposition. In discussing cutaneous vasculitis of the legs the role of cold exposure in increasing the viscosity of the blood and of gravity in distorting blood vessels, and thereby promoting turbulent flow patterns, is important.

The precise form the expression of the angiitis will take depends upon numerous factors including those which influence fibrin and platelet deposition and removal; additional elements such as the presence of ischemia or inflammatory by-products; whether the vessels involved are capillaries, veins or arteries; the relative activity of fibrinolysis and macrophage systems and those factors which determine whether the infiltrate will be primarily neutrophilic, eosinophilic or lymphocytic. The extent to which these and other as yet undiscovered factors are independent or interdependent will also be of importance in determining the clinical manifestations of the cutaneous angiitis.

Methods of proper therapy, like the problems of etiology and classification, remain unsettled. Some authors[19] advocate prompt and vigorous adminstration of systemic steroids, while others believe that such therapy is of no value; and, indeed, there is some evidence,[20,21] that preceding steroid therapy has, upon occasion, given rise to necrotizing vasculitis. Winkelmann[22] advocates steroid or ACTH therapy in fulminating acute vasculitis, but thinks that it is not indicated in the more subacute or chronic cases.

By way of illustrating some of the clinical variations seen in necrotizing vasculitis, we present brief summaries of four cases we studied.

Case Report 1. M.B., a 17-year-old male, was first seen in October 1964, at which time he gave the following history: Three years previously an ulcerated lesion appeared on his great toe, became infected, and then healed with application of unknown salves. Over the ensuing three years similar lesions had come and gone, usually one or two being present at any given time. Two months previously he had developed several lesions on his right ankle which yielded *Staphylococcus aureus* on culture. He was treated with numerous medicaments, including soaks, systemic and local antibiotics, and commercial staph toxoid. One month later an autogenous staph vaccine was prepared and administered by injection to the patient. Several weeks later numerous new lesions appeared on his left leg, feet, and buttocks. He also had developed swelling of his left knee and both ankles. He denied any other systemic symptomatology. He had had "rose fever" for the preceding year; his mother had asthma. Physical examination revealed hemorrhagic erythematous papules and patches varying from 0.5 to 10.0 cm. in diameter, primarily over the buttocks, elbows, and legs. Some lesions were ulcerated and had black eschars. Biopsy of a cutaneous lesion was reported as showing toxic vasculitis. Deep muscle biopsy showed no evidence of periarteritis nodosa. Other laboratory studies, including W.B.C., differential, Hct, sedimentation rate, BUN, creatinine, liver function tests, S.T.S., serum protein electrophoresis, cryoglobulins, antistreptolysin O titer, C-reactive protein, tuberculin and fungal skin tests, were normal. Skin tests to his own W.B.C., R.B.C., and animal DNA were negative. EKG, chest x-ray, upper and lower G.I. series were normal. Bacterial culture of a lesion grew streptococci, staphylococci, and *C. albicans*.

Therapy consisted of bacitracin ointment and Lassar's paste with 3 percent vioform locally and Aristocort 20 mg. daily by mouth. He was discharged improved, and his lesions continued to resolve slowly. In early 1965, he was lost to follow-up.

This boy is a fascinating example of necrotizing vasculitis (Fig. 3-5), particularly because his cutaneous lesions may represent a Shwartzman reaction. In this instance, the *Staphylococcus aureus* present in his ulcers or the commercial staph toxoid injections would function as the "primary" antigens to "prepare" his skin, and the autogenous vaccine would represent the "eliciting" injection.

Case Report 2. F.M., a 46-year-old male, in early 1963 noted several pustules on his legs which were treated with compresses and pHisohex scrubs. The lesions improved in two weeks but then recurred three weeks later, and on this occasion the same therapy was not effective. He was hospitalized in February 1963, at which time he showed anemia, weight loss, ankle edema, an ulcer of the tongue, and several sharply demarcated erythematous lesions over the left calf and right

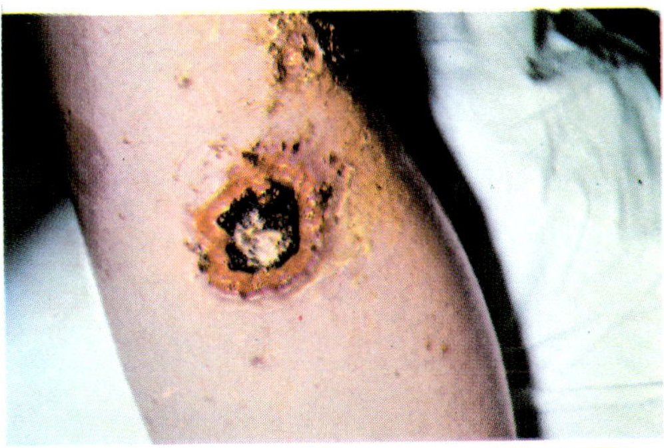

Fig. 3-5. Necrotizing vasculitis in Case Report 1. The hemorrhagic appearance is the salient feature.

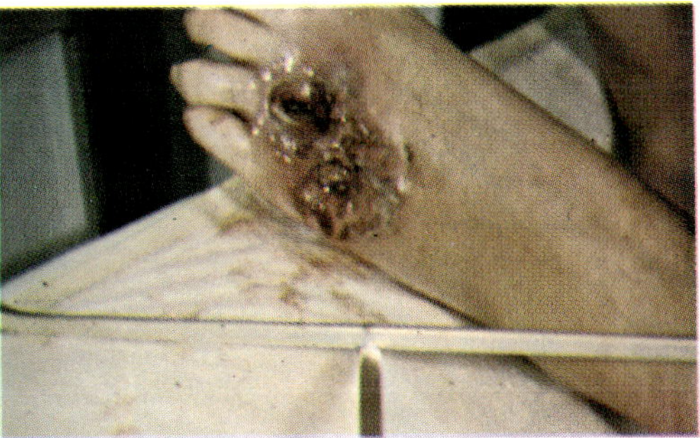

Fig. 3-6. Necrotizing vasculitis (pyoderma gangrenosum). Note the severe destructive process of the lesion in Case Report 3.

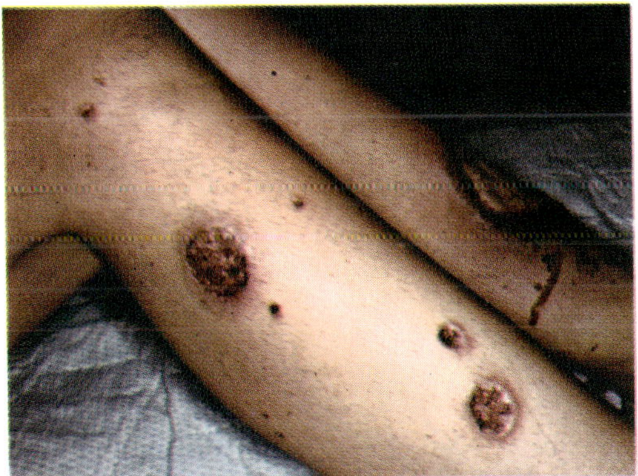

Fig. 3-7. Necrotizing vasculitis in Case Report 4.

ankle. After diagnostic studies and therapeutic measures, he was discharged but continued to have recurrent and persistent purulent lesions which had become more extensive, involving his hands, arms, and face, accompanied by painless swelling of the fingers. He also continued to exhibit ankle edema. On readmission to the hospital in May 1964, he had numerous punched-out, ulcerated crusted lesions ranging up to two centimeters in diameter, located primarily over the distal portions of the extremities, with a few on his buttocks. Numerous pustules were present over his back. He had marked ankle edema and also manifested edema of his fingers. An ulcerated crusted lesion (1 x 1 cm.), was noted on his left buccal mucosa. The remainder of his physical examination was unremarkable. Laboratory studies revealed a moderate hypochromic anemia, increased platelets, mild leukocytosis, moderate elevation of the $alpha_1$, $alpha_2$, and gamma globulins and guaiac positive stools. Numerous other studies were normal or negative, including his S.T.S., L.E. preps, urinalysis, latex fixation, uric acid, BUN, fungal skin tests, and cryoglobulins. Cultures of the skin lesions grew enterococci and *S. aureus*. Culture of the skin for tubercle bacilli and fungi was negative. X-rays of the hands and bones showed a bizarre picture with much periosteal proliferation, soft tissue swelling of the bones of the hands and feet, and cystic areas of bone resorption near joints. Bone marrow aspiration revealed hyperplasia of the myeloid series without evidence of leukemia or myeloma. Proctoscopy revealed polypoid masses which were believed to be pyogenic granulomas on biopsy. Skin biopsy showed a vasculitis.

On conservative therapy of compresses, topical steroid cream, and Terramycin orally, he improved. Following his discharge from the hospital, he experienced two recurrences of the leg lesions after the administration of aspirin. He has remained free of leg lesions since the drug has been discontinued.

In this patient the role played by aspirin is significant.

Case Report 3. F.W., a 44-year-old female, had experienced five severe episodes of pyoderma gangrenosum in the past fourteen years (Fig. 3-6). Before then she had suffered from ulcerative colitis for several years, and her initial attack of pyoderma gangrenosum in 1952 coincided with a flare of her colitis. Her second attack in 1956 followed her first pregnancy and was attributed to nutritional deficiency and a mild reactivation of the ulcerative colitis. She then remained free of lesions for the next seven years. Since July 1963, she had experienced three bouts of pyoderma gangrenosum, but had no gastrointestinal symptomatology. On these last three occasions her condition had required hospitalization for several weeks at a time. During one of the episodes she developed a urinary tract infection due to *E. coli* which cleared on antibiotic therapy. The lesions of pyoderma gangrenosum were not influenced by the antibiotics, and steroid therapy was required to control the cutaneous vasculitis. Repeated cultures of material from early bullous lesions showed no growth; serum protein electrophoresis revealed slight elevation of the beta globulin and a slight depression of the gamma globulin fractions; L.E. clot tests were negative on many occasions; chest x-ray and barium enema were within normal limits. Skin tests to the patient's own plasma, white and red blood cells were negative.

The cutaneous vasculitis of this patient could have been based on a Shwartzman phenomenon, as though she were a patient with a "prepared" skin, presumably reacting on two occasions to her ulcerative colitis, and on three occasions to as yet undefined antigens.

It is significant that the first episode of cutaneous vasculitis cleared when the ulcerative colitis was controlled; the second attack responded to an ulcerative colitis regimen combined with gamma globulin and short-term steroid therapy. The third and fourth episodes required higher steroid doses for longer periods of time, and the fifth attack responded to steroids fortified with chloroquine. This combination of drugs proved highly effective; after two months all medication was discontinued. She has remained free of symptoms to date.

Case Report 4. J.S., a 59-year-old male, was first seen in September 1963. He gave a history that six months previously he had noted flat, red macules on the anterior aspects of his legs and one on his scrotum. The lesions increased in size over a three-week period, became bullous, then ruptured, expelling blood and pus. An eschar formed four weeks later, and the lesions remained stationary. Subsequently he developed similar lesions on his arms and buttocks. He was treated elsewhere for five weeks with penicillin without improvement, then hospitalized and treated with chloromycetin for nine weeks which caused a profound anemia necessitating four transfusions. While receiving the chloromycetin he developed no new lesions.

Significant points in his past history were that he underwent a colectomy for carcinoma of the bowel in 1955, and four years later a partial resection of the right lung was performed for a solitary metastasis.

At the time of his initial visit in 1963, he was admitted to the University of Pennsylvania Hospital for diagnostic studies. At that time physical examination revealed hypertrophied, bluish-red and friable gums, an enlarged, hard, nonnodular liver, an indurated epididymis with a draining sinus, and numerous granulomatous crusting lesions of the arms and legs (Fig. 3-7). Laboratory studies revealed a mild leukocytosis, an elevated sedimentation rate, and hypergammaglobulinemia. Numerous other studies were normal. Culture of the skin lesions for bacteria, fungi, and tubercle bacilli was negative. Three biopsies were taken: one showed only nonspecific dermatitis, another granulomatous tissue, and the third vasculitis. Tissue specimens from the scrotal lesions were cultured, and a fungus was recovered which was believed to be *Blastomyces*.

Local x-ray therapy and intralesional triamcinolone were tried, but produced no change in the lesions. The granulomatous lesions healed slowly on a regimen of pHisohex scrubs and neosporin ointment. About one month after discharge, he developed erythematous fluctuant nodules on his right lower leg, which did not have any features of necrotizing vasculitis and which resolved on soaks and neosporin cream. He remained free of lesions for the next 18 months and then suffered a fatal myocardial infarction.

We have no explanation for the cause of vasculitis in this patient. Of significance, however, was the fact that improvement in the skin lesions followed cessation of all oral and parenteral antibiotic therapy; improvement was attained with institution of simple topical measures.

In summary, the medical literature abounds with classifications, clinical syndromes and histologic features of the various cutaneous expressions of vasculitis. However, these entities are in a confused and changing etiologic, diagnostic, and therapeutic state, and it would seem unwise at this point to attempt arbitrary and perhaps artificial classifications. At the present time, in our opinion, recognition of the underlying factor of vasculitis is the crucial finding, irrespective of the precise form of its clinical expression.

References

1. Zeek, P.M.: Periarteritis nodosa and other forms of necrotizing angiitis. New Eng. J. Med., *248*:764, 1953.

2. Copeman, P.W.M., and Ryan, T.J.: The problems of classification of cutaneous angiitis with reference to histopathology and pathogenesis. *In* The microvascular system of the skin. Brit. J. Derm. *82*:2, Suppl. No. 5, 1970

3. McCombs, R.P.: Systemic "allergic" vasculitis. JAMA, *194*: 1059, 1965.

4. Winkelmann, R.K., and Ditto, W.B.: Cutaneous and visceral syndromes of necrotizing or "allergic" angiitis: A study of 38 cases. Medicine, *43*: 59, 1964.

5. O'Duffy, J.D., Scherbel, A.L., Reidbord, H.E., and McCormack, L.J.: Necrotizing angiitis: I.A clinical review of twenty-seven autopsied cases. Cleveland Clin. Quart., *32*: 87, 1965.

6. Alarcon-Segovia, D., and Brown, A.L., Jr.: Classification and etiologic aspects of necrotizing angiitides: an analytic approach to a confused subject with a critical review of the evidence for hypersensitivity in polyarteritis nodosa. Proc. Mayo Clinic, *39*: 205, 1964.

7. Winkelmann, R.K.: Diagnosis and treatment of allergic angiitis (anaphylactoid purpura). Postgrad. Med., *27*: 437, 1960.

8. McCarthy, J.T.: Cutaneous vasculitis. Med. Clin. N. America, *49*:761, 1965.

9. Champion, R.H., and Wilkinson, D.S.: Affecting blood vessels. *In* Rook, A.J., Wilkinson, D.S., and Ebling, F.J.G. (eds.): Textbook of Dermatology. Oxford, Blackwell Scientific Publications, 1968.

10. Borrie, P., and Stansfeld, A.: Cutaneous vasculitis. *In* Mackenna, R.M.B.: Modern Trends in Dermatology, p. 167. London, Butterworths, 1966.

11. Copeman, P.W.M., and Ryan, T.J.: The problems of classification of cutaneous angiitis with reference to histopathology and pathogenesis. *In* The microvascular system of the skin. Brit. J. Derm., *82*: 2, Suppl. No. 5, 1970.

12. Citron, B.P., *et al.*: Necrotizing angiitis associated with drug abuse. New Eng. J. Med., *283*:1003, 1970.

13. Winkelmann, R.K.: Diagnosis and treatment of allergic angiitis (anaphylactoid purpura). Postgrad. Med., *27*: 437, 1960.

14. Hjort, P.F., and Rapaport, S.I.: The Shwartzman reaction: pathogenetic mechanisms and clinical manifestations. Ann. Rev. Med., *16*: 135, 1965.

15. Binkley, G.W.: Dermatitis nodularis necrotica. Arch. Derm., *75*: 387, 1957.

16. Goldgraber, M.B., and Kirsner, J.B.: Gangrenous skin lesions associated with chronic ulcerative colitis. Gastroenterology, *39*: 94, 1960.

17. Samitz, M.H.: Cutaneous vasculitis in assocation with ulcerative colitis. Cutis, *2*:383, 1966.

18. Copeman, P.W.M., and Ryan, T.J.: The problems of classification of cutaneous angiitis with reference to histopathology and pathogenesis. *In* The microvascular system of the skin. Brit. J. Derm. *82*:2, Suppl. No. 5, 1970.

19. McCombs, R.P.: Systemic "allergic" vasculitis. JAMA, *194*: 1059, 1965.

20. Johnson, R.L., *et al.*: Steroid therapy and vascular lesions in rheumatoid arthritis. Arthritis Rheum. *2*: 224, 1959.

21. O'Quinn, S.E., Kennedy, C.B., and Baker, DeW.T.: Peripheral vascular lesions in rheumatoid arthritis. Arch. Derm., *92*: 489, 1965.

22. Winkelmann, R.K.: Diagnosis and treatment of allergic angiitis (anaphylactoid purpura). Postgrad. Med., *27*: 437, 1960.

Figs. 3-8, 9, 10, 11, 12, 13. The diversity of lesions in cutaneous vasculitis is broad; hemor-

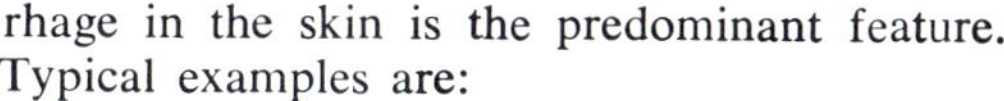

rhage in the skin is the predominant feature. Typical examples are:

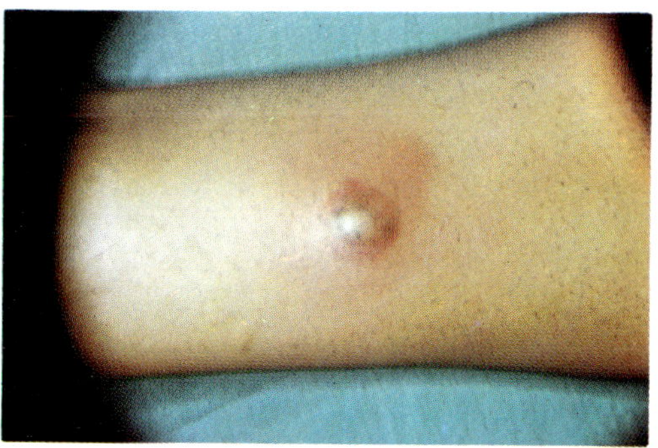

Fig. 3-8. Close-up of an early inflammatory lesion (24 hours old) of pyoderma gangrenosum. The pronounced bluish-red areola is characteristic.

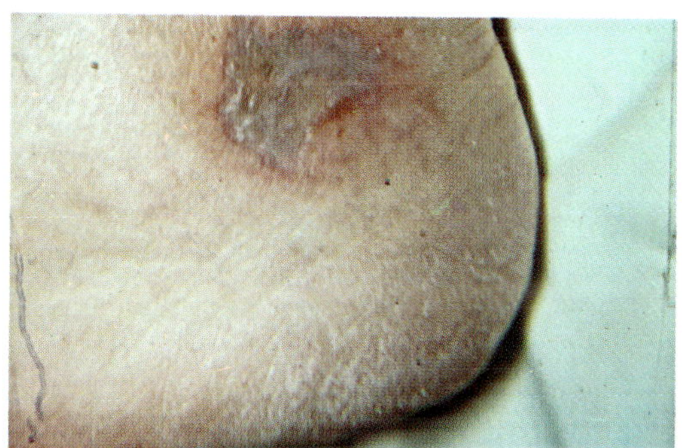

Fig. 3-9. Close-up of an early lesion (2 days old). The intensely hemorrhagic necrotizing reaction is a constant salient clinical feature.

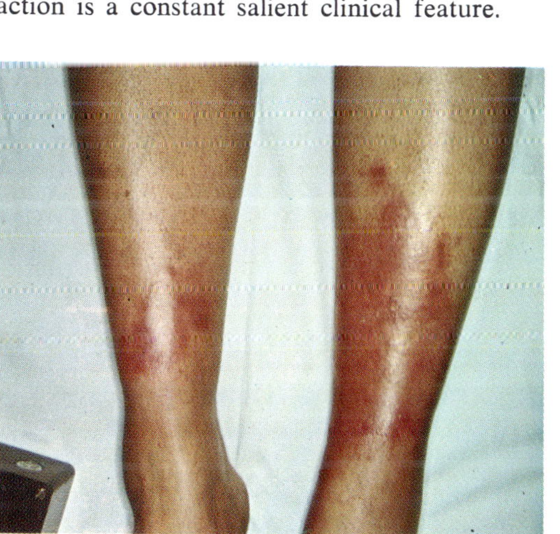

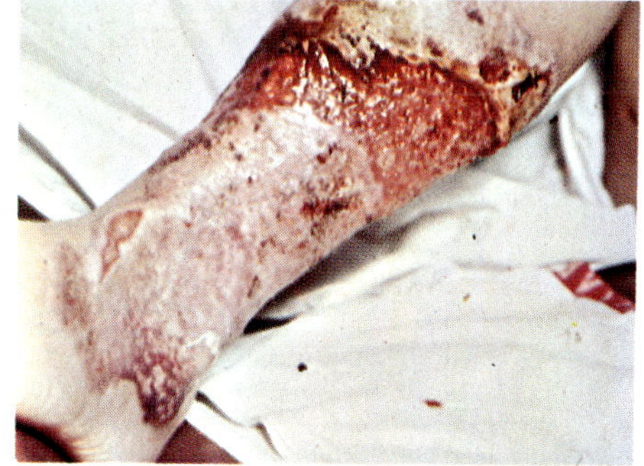

Fig. 3-11. Severe phagedenic ulceration in patient with pyoderma gangrenosum in association with ulcerative colitis.

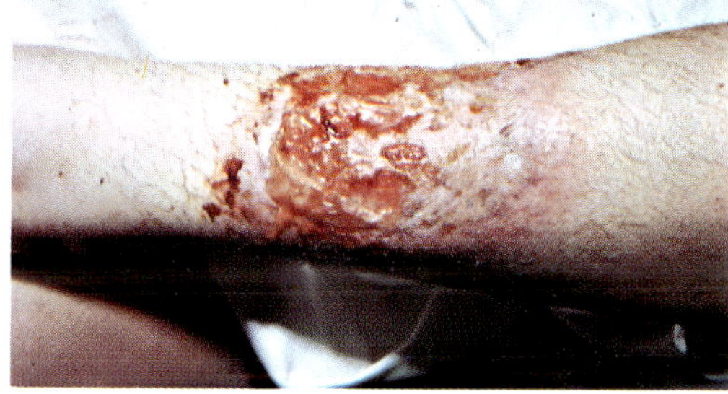

Fig. 3-12. Necrotizing ulceration complicating Crohn's disease in a 19-year-old girl.

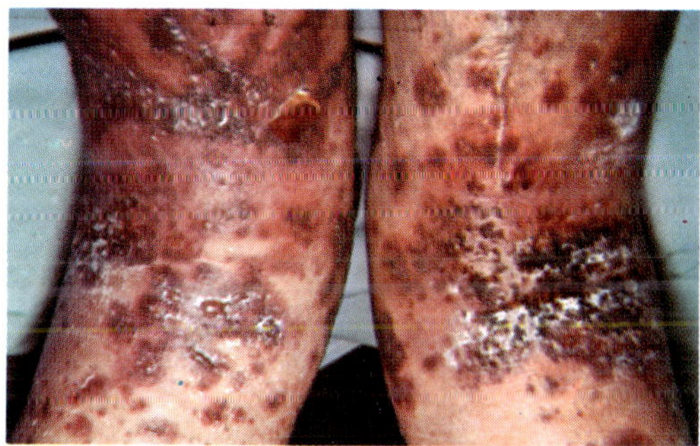

Fig. 3-13. Severe necrotizing vasculitis in a patient with systemic lupus erythematosus.

Fig. 3-10. Early lesions presenting as a broad mat of erythema. The lesions broke down subsequently into extensive ulcerations.

LIVEDO RETICULARIS

Livedo reticularis is a physical sign which may indicate significant systemic disease or may be purely local. The disorder presents as a purplish, permanent, mottled vascular pattern, usually occurring on the lower extremity, but also occasionally appearing on the buttocks, arms or trunk. In the past there has been much confusion concerning the significance of livedo reticularis because of a failure to recognize livedo as a cutaneous sign associated with a variety of systemic disorders. Adequate studies should be made in each patient with this condition to rule out a systemic etiology.

Renaut in 1883 and Unna in 1896 postulated that the arterial supply to the skin was arranged in cones 1 to 3 cm. in diameter. An area of anastomosis with neighboring cones was assumed to occur at the periphery of each cone. In these areas a relatively diminished blood supply was believed to exist. Anatomical investigation has failed to demonstrate any such pattern of the cutaneous vessels. However skin temperature studies tend to support its presence.

The basic mechanism of production of livedo is dilation of the minute vessels of the subpapillary venous plexus with subsequent marked slowing of blood flow. At times the blood flow may actually cease or even reverse direction and thrombosis may occur. The resultant ischemia outlines the anastomotic areas between the cones as a violaceous reticulated network. Clinical observation confirms that the darker areas are relatively ischemic; in those patients with livedo reticularis who develop ulceration, the ulcers always originate in the dark areas.

Physiological Forms of Livedo Reticularis

Cutis Marmorata. This is a physiological response to cold seen in the majority of normal children and is of no significance. It may be seen in some adults, particularly in women, and is more prominent in the presence of debilitating illness. This condition has been reported in cases of perniosis in association with acrocyanosis and erythrocyanosis and has resulted in ulcerations, particularly during the winter months.

Pathological Causes of Livedo Reticularis

Perniosis. This is often associated with mottling of the skin; the mechanism of this response of the blood vessels to cold is unknown.

Arteriosclerosis. This may, in unusual instances, be associated with livedo reticularis.

Polyarteritis Nodosa. This condition is associated with livedo at times; however, a widespread or patchy livedo, though suggestive of polyarteritis, is not as diagnostic as previously thought. The majority of cases associated with polyarteritis nodosa also have nodules. The diagnosis of polyarteritis should be confirmed by deep biopsy and histological demonstration of a panarteritis which distinguishes it from

CAUSES OF LIVEDO RETICULARIS (adapted from Champion[1])

- I. Physiological
  - A. Cutis marmorata
- II. Pathological
  - A. Perniosis
  - B. Arteriosclerosis
  - C. Arteritis
    1. polyarteritis nodosa
    2. lupus erythematosus
    3. dermatomyositis
    4. rheumatoid arteritis
    5. rheumatic fever
    6. syphilis
    7. tuberculosis
    8. pancreatitis
    9. mycosis fungoides
  - D. Intravascular occlusion
    1. arterial emboli
    2. thrombocythemia
    3. cryoglobulinemia
  - E. Congenital livedo
  - F. Idiopathic

---

other conditions associated with livedo in which the pathology is mainly an endarteritis.

Bard and Winkelmann[2] have described a segmental hyalinizing vasculitis which presents as ulcerative disease of the legs, the ulcerations developing in a reticular pattern. The typical mottling of livedo reticularis is absent; however, the pattern of ulceration so resembles that seen in livedo reticularis at times, that the condition has been described as "Livedo reticularis with ulcerations without livedo reticularis." This disorder is now considered a separate entity and has been named livedo vasculitis. Interestingly, the scars resulting from this disorder clinically resemble atrophie blanche, although they differ from it histologically.

Lupus Erythematosus. There are two mechanisms by which mottling may occur with lupus erythematosus. A true vasculitis may occur which may be associated with severe ulcerations and necrosis. Alternatively, the typical cruption of lupus erythematosus may become manifest in the partially ischemic areas of the livedo pattern.

Thrombocythemia. Champion and Rook[3] reported three cases of thrombocythemia presenting with circumscribed areas of livedo and gangrene of single toes. The livedo of thrombocythemia may be reversible and clear with prompt treatment. Early recognition of this condition may preclude later development of hemorrhage and thrombosis which is sure to occur if treatment is delayed.

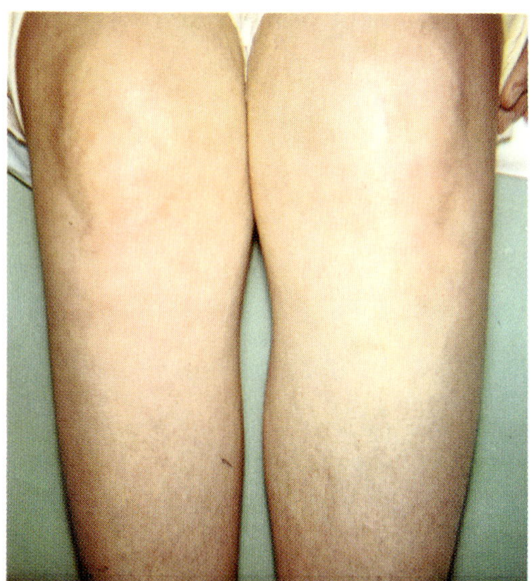

Fig. 3-14. Livedo reticularis in association with cryoglobulinemia.

Miscellaneous Diseases. In rare instances, a number of other disorders, including dermatomyositis, rheumatoid arteritis, syphilis, tuberculosis, mycosis fungoides and arterial emboli have been associated with livedo reticularis. Localized areas of livedo may result from the intravascular precipitation of serum proteins. We have followed a case of severe cryoglobulinemia. The initial presenting symptom was livedo reticularis (Fig. 3-14); subsequently, classical lesions of necrotizing vasculitis developed. On immunofluorescence of the vasculitis lesions, deposits of immunoglobulins of the same classes as those found in the cryoglobulins were detected. Sigmund and Shelley[4] reported a case of pancreatitis associated with a patch of livedo reticularis of the abdominal wall apparently due to vascular damage from pancreatic enzymes.

Congenital Livedo. This term is reserved for a relatively rare group of cases in which an irregular mottling is present at birth. It may be confined to one limb or be generalized. It is quite prominent in appearance and the skin may be atrophic. Although some fading may occur in time, the eruption is likely to persist indefinitely. Systemic involvement has not been reported. It is likely that this represents a developmental anomaly.

Idiopathic Livedo Reticularis. A large group of patients may be seen in which no associated cause may be found. They are frequently women in the 25 to 45 year age group. Unlike the patchy asymmetrical livedo in patients with arteritis, this type is more likely to be diffuse. The condition is often progressive and increasing ischemia of the skin may lead to disabling ulceration. Usually this is worse in winter, but in a number of cases the ulcers appear during the summer and are preceded by edema.

A small minority of the idiopathic cases do have widespread arterial disease and may have cerebral thromboses, intermittent claudication, angina pectoris and even renal involvement. Although there is no

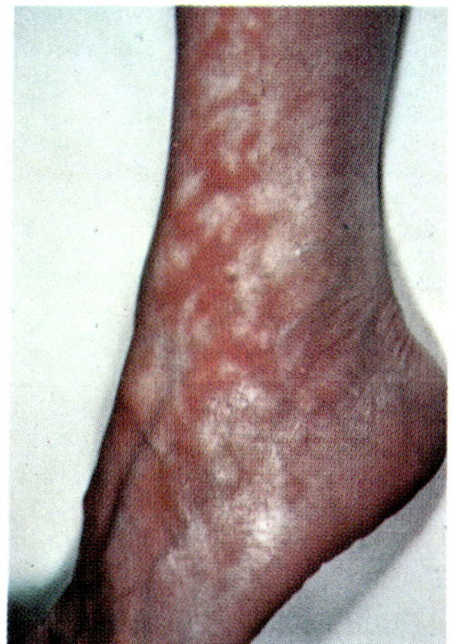

Fig. 3-15. Erythema ab igne. This disorder caused by repeated exposure to moderate heat may at times be confused with livedo reticularis.

effective treatment for those cases with systemic involvement, the cases with only skin involvement may be helped with prolonged anticoagulant therapy.

The histology of the cases, with or without systemic disease, is similar. The pathological changes are confined to the intima which is greatly thickened so that it may obliterate the lumen of the vessel. Some thickening of the media may be present, but there are no inflammatory changes.

Livedo reticularis may at times be confused with *erythema ab igne*. In this disorder, repeated exposure to moderate heat will cause a reticulate erythema and later pigmentation which becomes apparent after about two weeks. More severe exposure may lead to bulla formation and squamous cell carcinoma has been reported in areas of prolonged exposure. The most common sites for this condition are the inner and outer aspects of the shins (Fig. 3-15) and in men the lesions may occur over the knees where the clothes are in direct contact with the skin. Other areas affected are frequently due to the application of hot water bottles, heating pads and the like.

The clinical diagnosis of livedo reticularis is not difficult. The important point to be emphasized is that the recognition of the cutaneous pattern should alert the physician to investigate the patient to determine whether significant systemic disease is present.

References

1. Champion, R. H.: Livedo reticularis: a review. Brit. J. Derm., *77*: 167, Apr., 1965.

2. Bard, J. W., and Winkelmann, R. K.: Livedo vasculitis. Segmental hyalinizing vasculitis of the dermis. Arch. Derm., *96*: 489, Nov., 1967.

3. Champion, R. H., and Rook, A.: Idiopathic thrombocythemia. Arch. Derm., *87*: 302, 1963.

4. Sigmund, W. J., and Shelley, W. B.: Cutaneous manifestations of acute pancreatitis, with special reference to livedo reticularis. New Eng. J. Med., *251*: 851, Nov., 1954.

PIGMENTED PURPURIC DERMATOSES

The differential diagnosis of purpura occurring on the legs embraces a wide spectrum of disease states. The pigmented purpuric eruptions, though somewhat uncommon, are by no means rare; frequently, however, they are not recognized by the general physician. If a pigmented purpuric dermatosis is suspected clinically, then a comparatively few screening tests are indicated to rule out other forms of purpura and to establish the diagnosis. A simple classification is presented in Table 3-1.

Originally each of the pigmented purpuric dermatoses was described as a separate entity because the authors considered the clinical morphology of the eruption to be distinctive. Additional observations, however, raised questions about the uniqueness of each of these dermatoses (Figs. 3-16, 3-17, 3-18).

Although theoretically each of the pigmented purpuric eruptions is quite distinctive, clinically often there are not enough characteristic features to distinguish one from another.[1] Common features in the pigmented purpuric dermatoses are shown in Tables 3-2, 3-3, and 3-4. The eczematid-like purpura of Doucas and Kapetanakis, itching purpura

Table 3-1. Pigmented Purpuric Dermatoses of the Lower Extremities

I. COMMON
   A. Schamberg's progressive pigmentary dermatosis
      1. Eczematid-like purpura of Doucas and Kapetanakis
      2. Itching purpura of Loewenthal
      3. Transitory pigmented purpuric eruption of the lower extremities (Osment *et al.*)
   B. Majocchi's purpura annularis telangiectodes

II. INFREQUENT
   A. Pigmented purpuric lichenoid dermatitis of Gougerot-Blum
   B. Angioma serpiginosum of Hutchinson

III. MORPHOLOGICALLY SIMILAR BUT ETIOLOGICALLY UNRELATED*
   A. Hyperglobulinemic purpura of Waldenstrom
   B. Stasis dermatitis

*Not usually included in etiologic classifications of pigmented purpuric eruptions.

Table 3-2. Four Classical Pigmented Purpuric Dermatoses of the Lower Extremities

FEATURES IN COMMON:
1. Etiology: unknown
2. Hematologic studies: normal
3. Course: chronic
4. Prognosis: benign
5. Histology: capillaritis (angioma serpiginosum controversial)

DIFFERENCES:
1. Morphology: variable

Table 3-3. Hyperglobulinemic Purpura

FEATURES IN COMMON WITH PIGMENTED DERMATOSES:
1. Course: chronic
2. Prognosis: benign
3. Morphology

DIFFERENCES:
1. Etiology: presumably different, related to hyperglobulinemia
2. Hematologic abnormalities
   (a) elevated gamma globulin
   (b) elevated sedimentation rate
   (c) anemia

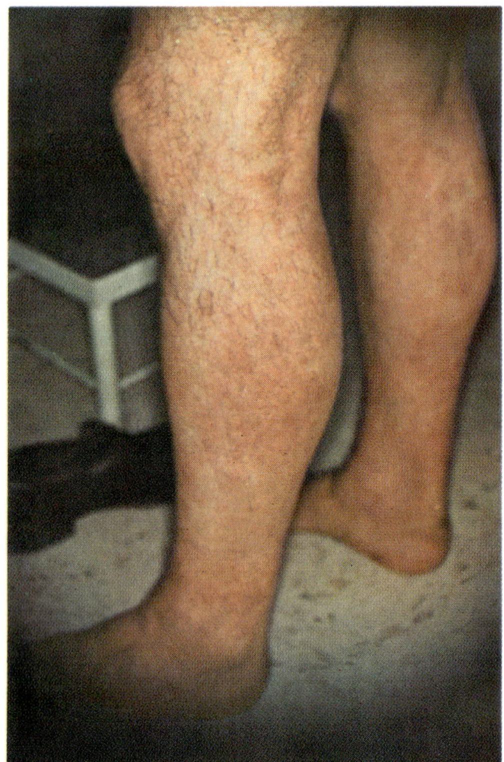

Fig. 3-16. Pigmented purpuric dermatosis (Schamberg's).

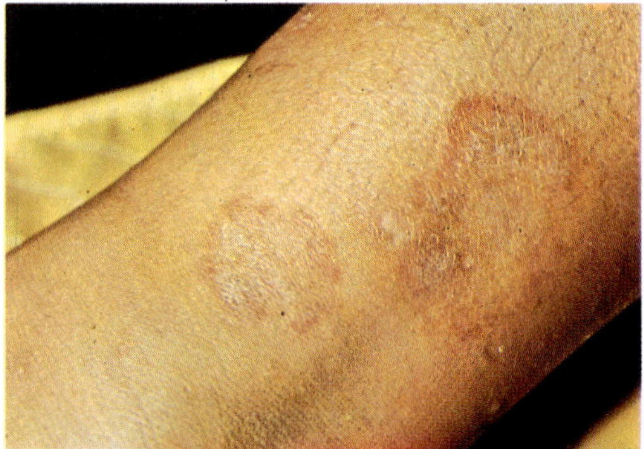

Fig. 3-17. Pigmented purpuric dermatosis (Majocchi's purpura annularis telangiectodes).

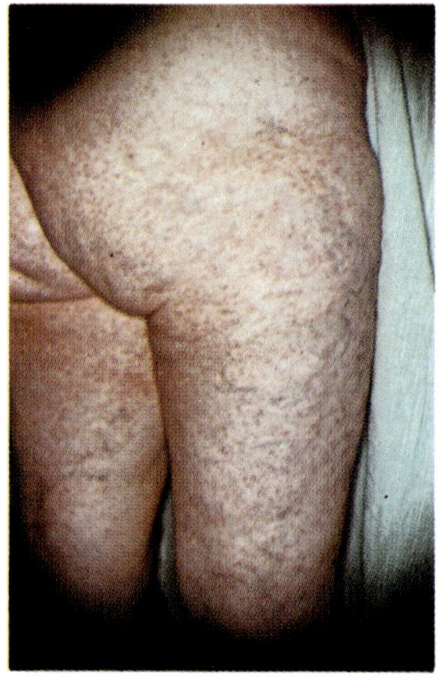

Fig. 3-18. Pigmented purpuric dermatosis (Gougerot-Blum).

of Loewenthal, and transitory pigmented purpuric eruption of the lower extremities have been included under Schamberg's disease in Tables 3-1 and 3-4 because many dermatologists regard them as merely atypical cases of Schamberg's disease.

The microscopic changes consist essentially of a chronic capillaritis with swelling, degeneration, and proliferation of the endothelial cells, extravasation of erythrocytes and a pericapillary lymphocytic infiltrate in the upper dermis.[2] Hemosiderin also may be found. The net result is capillary fragility resulting in purpura and pigmentation.

The general consensus at present is that the separation of these four eruptions into distinct diagnostic entities is unwarranted. However, Barker and Sachs pointed out that the pigment, purpura, inflammatory changes, and histologic findings of a vasculitis seen in varying degrees in Majocchi's, Schamberg's, and Gougerot and Blum's dermatoses are not present in angioma serpiginosum. The authors consider angioma serpiginosum to be a "minute vascular neoplasm of angiomatous or

Table 3-4. Differential Diagnosis of Purpuric Eruptions

	Schamberg's disease	*Majocchi's dermatosis*	*Dermatitis of Gougerot and Blum*	*Angioma serpiginosum*	*Hyperglobulinemic purpura*
Primary lesion	"Cayenne pepper" punctum	Punctum due to capillary ectasia	Reddish papule	Angiomatous papular punctum	Pinhead petechia
Age at onset	Adults	Adults	Adults	80% before age 20	Adults
Sex	Males 5:1 [a]	More frequent in females	More frequent in males	Females 9:1	Females 3:1
Distribution	Legs unilateral	Legs bilateral symmetrical	Legs bilateral symmetrical	Legs unilateral(?)	Legs bilateral symmetrical
Purpura	+	+	± / +	0	++
Pigmentation	+++	+	+ (?)	0	+
Telangiectasia	0	++	0 / +	+	0
Pruritus	0 [b]	0	++	+	0
Lab. studies [c]	Normal	Normal	Normal	Normal	Normal [d]

[a] Exceptions: Itching purpura, equal sex incidence; transitory pigmented purpuric eruption, equal sex incidence.

[b] Exceptions: Itching purpura, significant pruritus; transitory pigmented purpuric eruption, mild pruritus.

[c] Normal studies include: Hgb., Hct., W.B.C., differential, platelet count, bleeding time, clotting time. Tourniquet test positive in 50-75% of cases of each dermatosis.

[d] Abnormal blood findings: Elevated gamma globulin and erythrocyte sedimentation rate; anemia.

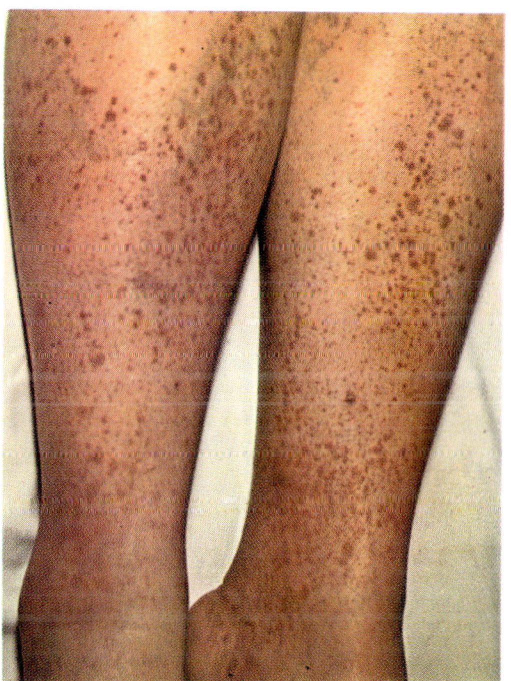

Fig. 3-19. Hyperglobulinemic purpura of Waldenstrom.

telangiectatic nature" and would classify it as a "nevoid condition or form of vascular nevus."[3]

Therapy for all of the dermatoses is empiric and symptomatic. Since the eruptions are benign, if any form of therapy is attempted, it should be very conservative. Variable results have been reported with ascorbic acid, bland antipruritic emollients, and fluocinolone acetonide cream with Saran wrap occlusion.[4] Clearing of the cutaneous lesions has been reported following the systemic administration of corticosteroids,[5] but there would not seem to be any valid reason for the institution of such therapy in these banal disorders.

IDIOPATHIC HYPERGLOBULINEMIC PURPURA

Waldenstrom in 1943 introduced an entity characterized by chronic purpura of the legs appearing in recurrent attacks over many years, an elevated serum gamma globulin with a normal albumin content, and an elevated erythrocyte sedimentation rate.[6] The majority of cases are female. A mild to moderate normochromic normocytic anemia, which is refractory to therapy, is usually present. Bleeding studies are normal. Pruritus is usually absent.[7] Clinically the disease has some similarities to multiple myeloma from which it must be distinguished, since hyperglobulinemic purpura is usually a benign disorder. Rarely do patients with hyperglobulinemic purpura develop multiple myeloma.[8,9] Other systemic disease states associated with an elevated gamma globulin and purpura (e.g., lupus erythematosus, sarcoid and Sjögren's syndrome) must be excluded.[10] After repeated showers of purpuric lesions over a period of years, the skin of the legs may show residual mottled brownish pigmentation, which probably represents hemosiderin deposits (Fig. 3-19). The purpuric eruption of hyperglobulinemic purpura may thus mimic the pigmented purpuric dermatoses; the possibility exists, as pointed out by Goltz and Good,[11] that some persons may have been incorrectly classified as having one of the pigmented dermatoses when analysis of their serum proteins might reveal that they have hyperglobulinemic purpura.

STASIS DERMATITIS

The morphologic picture of stasis hemosiderosis is often clinically identical with the picture seen in the pigmented purpuric eruptions. Infrared photography and the presence of venous incompetence would help to separate stasis from other conditions.

Stasis dermatitis is discussed more completely on pages 68-72.

References

1. Randall, S. J., Kierland, R. R., and Montgomery, H.: Pigmented purpuric eruptions. Arch. Derm. Syph., *64*: 177, 1951.

2. Lever, W. F.: Histopathology of the Skin. ed. 3, p. 164, Philadelphia, J. B. Lippincott, 1961.

3. Barker, L. P., and Sachs, P. M.: Angioma serpiginosum. Arch. Derm., *92*: 613, 1965.

4. Freedman, R., Hirsch, P., and Becker, S. W.: Treatment of two cases of itching purpura. Arch. Derm., *87*: 740, 1963.

5. Osment, L. S., *et al.*: Transitory pigmented purpuric eruption of the lower extremities, Arch. Derm., *81*: 591, 1960.

6. Taylor, F. E., and Battle, J. D., Jr.: Benign hyperglobulinemic purpura: case report. Ann. Int. Med., *40*: 350, 1954.

7. Hambrick, G. W., Jr.: Dysproteinemic purpura of the hypergammaglobulinemic type. Arch. Derm., *77*:23, 1958.

8. Rogers, W. R., and Welch, J. D.: Purpura hyperglobulinemica terminating in multiple myeloma. Arch. Int. Med., *100*: 478, 1957.

9. Savin, R. C.: Hyperglobulinemic purpura terminating in myeloma, hyperlipemia and xanthomatosis. Arch. Derm., *92*: 679, 1965.

10. Seiden, G. E., and Wurzel, H. A.: Idiopathic benign hyperglobulinemic purpura. New Eng. J. Med., *255*: 170, 1956.

11. Goltz, R. W., and Good, R. A.: Benign hyperglobulinemic purpura. Arch. Derm., *83*: 26, 1961.

12. Doucas, C., and Kapetanakis, J.: Eczematid-like purpura. Dermatologica, *106*: 86, 1953.

13. Loewenthal, L. J. A.: Itching purpura. Brit. J. Derm., *66*: 95, 1954.

ATROPHIE BLANCHE

Atrophie blanche occurs predominantly in middle-aged women who have varicose veins either with or without stasis dermatitis. The patients develop small purpuric erythematous and edematous plaques with a hyperpigmented border and prominent telangiectatic vessels located on the lower third of the leg (Fig. 3-20).[1] The involved areas may undergo superficial but painful ulceration. In either case the lesions ultimately heal with formation of a white atrophic scar (Fig. 3-21). Histologic changes are characteristic and show thrombosis of small cutaneous arterioles with wedge-shaped infarction and eventual fibrosis of the overlying skin.[2]

References

1. Frain-Bell, W.: Atrophie blanche. Trans. St. John's Hosp. Derm. Soc., *42*: 59, 1959.

2. Gray, H. R. *et al.*: Atrophie blanche: periodic painful ulcers of lower extremities. Arch. Derm., *93*: 187, Feb. 1966.

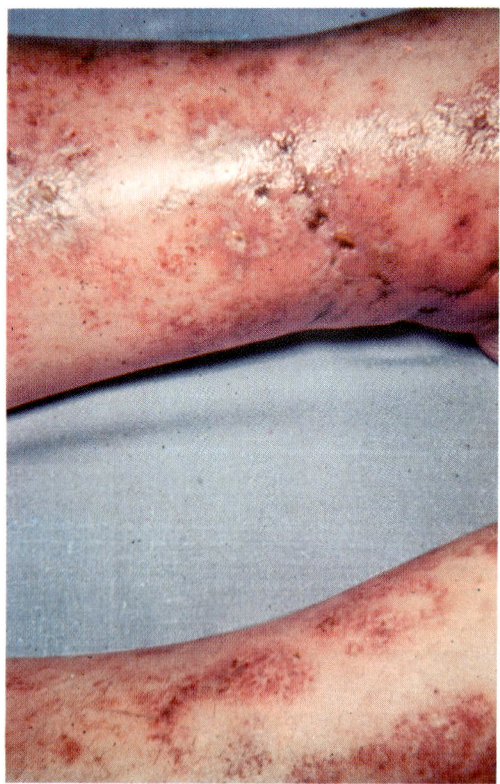

Fig. 3-20. Atrophie blanche. Early lesions.

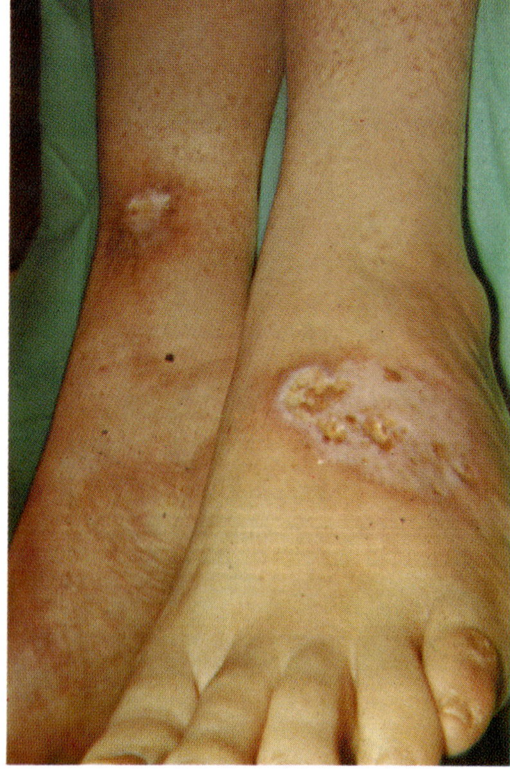

Fig. 3-21. Atrophie blanche. Note characteristic white scar.

4

Metabolic Disorders

DIABETES

There are no pathognomonic skin signs of diabetes, although some of the changes are sufficiently typical to alert the physician. The lower extremities are by far the most commonly affected skin areas in diabetes.

Cutaneous disorders complicating diabetes include pruritus, bacterial and fungal infections, pigmentation, xanthomatous lesions, and dermal changes secondary to vascular disease and neurotrophic disorders.

Pruritus

Pruritus is the most common symptom affecting the skin of the diabetic. While it may be generalized, it most commonly is localized to the legs. The most frequent cause is dryness or asteatosis of the skin which is promoted by excess washing with hot water and soap or by a decrease in the humidity, as occurs in winter. Decreased perspiration from impairment of cutaneous nerves may be an additional factor. Therapy consists of hydrating the skin. Bathe the skin in lukewarm water for 15 to 30 minutes and then apply a lubricating cream or ointment such as aqua and aquaphor (Eucerin), hydrophilic petrolatum, Vaseline or a hydrogenated vegetable oil (Crisco, Spry) over the wet skin. Increasing the water content of the air with a humidifier is also important. Hot water and soap should be minimized.

Cutaneous Infections

While it is recognized that diabetes mellitus increases the susceptibility of the skin to infection,[1] the mechanism responsible is unclear. Dehydration, abnormal cellular nutrition and an altered immunologic capacity are now considered causative factors rather than elevated tissue glucose levels.

Candidiasis (Moniliasis)

Recurrent or persistent cutaneous candidiasis may occasionally be the first sign or symptom of diabetes and should alert the clinician to investigate this possibility. Candidiasis is most likely to occur in the patient whose hyperglycemia is poorly controlled. Clinically, candidiasis presents as erythematous patches, often with scattered surrounding peripheral pustules, occurring primarily in intertriginous areas such as the perineum, medial aspects of the thighs, under the breasts, in the axillae or between folds of skin. It also occurs in the toe webs resulting in a macerated fissured pruritic eruption often misdiagnosed as ringworm. Moniliasis may also involve the toenails and paronychial tissues.

The clinical diagnosis is confirmed by observing budding yeasts and filaments in KOH mounts and by culturing the organism on Saboraud's agar.

Treatment consists of proper control of the diabetes, maintaining a dry, well-ventilated skin surface through the wearing of sandals, open shoes or shoes made of lightweight materials, use of an absorbent powder and by wearing absorbent cotton socks rather than stretch socks of nylon or other synthetic fibers. Compresses or soaks (Burow's solution, potassium permanganate) should be used in the acute phase. Specific anticandidal agents such as nystatin or amphotericin B should be applied sparingly but frequently. Though gentian violet also is effective, it is very messy, often hinders proper clinical evaluation because of its deep purple color and occasionally may irritate the involved skin.

Tinea Pedis

While the incidence of dermatophyte infections of the feet is probably no greater in diabetics than in nondiabetics, the disorder assumes much greater significance in the diabetic patient. Untreated or improperly treated, tinea pedis may lead to extensive bacterial secondary infection with cellulitis and the occasional development of septicemia, or to gangrene which may necessitate amputation.

Scrupulous care of the skin of the feet, maintaining ventilation and dryness, the use of absorbent socks and powder, and the wearing of ventilated shoes or sandals are mandatory.

The clinical and laboratory diagnosis of tinea pedis and its therapy are described in Chapter 2.

Bacterial Infections

It is usually thought that the incidence of pyodermas is greater in diabetics than in the general population.[2] There is no question that bacterial infections are much more serious in the diabetic. Such infections increase the insulin requirement and may precipitate diabetic acidosis. Diminished circulation and peripheral cutaneous diabetic neuropathy may also contribute to the severity of bacterial infections of the feet. Therapy consists of control of the diabetes, local soaks or compresses, topical and systemic antibiotics and proper foot care. Culture and sensitivity studies of the organism should be done to aid in selecting the proper antibiotic.

Skin Changes Due to Obliterative Arteriosclerosis

Arteriosclerotic changes of the blood vessels of the lower extremity occur more commonly, are more severe and have their onset earlier in diabetics. Signs and symptoms produced are due to the effects of tissue ischemia and may consist of pain after exercise or at rest, coldness of the feet, numbness, tingling or decreased tactile sensation, and atrophy of the skin and appendages (lack of hair and lack of sweating). A waxy pallor of the foot on elevation, with mottled bluish-red discoloration on dependency, accompanied by a delayed return of the color are virtually pathognomonic for occlusive arterial disease. If the pallor persists when the leg is dependent, even more severe arterial disease is indicated.

Large callosities or corns may form on the feet because of increased dryness of the skin from atrophy of the skin and sweat glands. Deep perforating ulcers (mal perforans) may develop in the calluses, especially on the ball of the foot (Figs. 4-1, 4-2).

Ulceration and gangrene often occur, usually beginning over the ankles, heels or toes, precipitated by trauma and infection (Fig. 4-3).

Therapy is generally unsatisfactory. Conservative topical therapy, good foot care and careful control of the diabetes are essential.

Diabetic Dermopathy

Melin[3] in 1964 and Binkley[4,5] shortly thereafter, described multiple discrete atrophic pigmented macular lesions occurring on the shins (Fig. 4-4). The lesions are usually asymptomatic and are incidental findings on physical examination. Binkley suggested the term "diabetic dermopathy"; Bauer *et al.*[6] in 1966 coined the term "pigmented pretibial patches" but Binkley's term has currency. The lesions occur most commonly in males over 30 years of age. Bauer *et al.* noted such lesions in 17 percent of adults with diabetes and 3 percent of adults without diabetes. Binkley relates the lesions to pathologic changes in the cutaneous blood vessels analogous to those in neuropathy, nephropathy and retinopathy. The lesions probably represent the result of minor trauma occurring in areas of cutaneous small vessel disease and may therefore not be specifically related to diabetes mellitus. No therapy is necessary.

Necrobiosis Lipoidica Diabeticorum

Necrobiosis lipoidica diabeticorum (NLD) was once thought to be a pathognomonic, though rare, sign of diabetes. It is now recognized that some persons with NLD have no clinical diabetes, though the possibility is often raised that they will eventually develop the disease. Glucose tolerance tests after ACTH may show a prediabetic pattern.

Necrobiosis lipoidica diabeticorum is a rare manifestation of diabetes, occurring in approximately 0.3 percent.[7] Its precise pathogenesis is unknown. It is clearly not related to the hyperglycemia or severity of the diabetes. Control of the diabetes has little effect on the skin lesions.

The lesions of NLD are atrophic, yellowish depressed areas with telangiectatic blood vessels coursing through them (Fig. 4-5 and Fig. 4-6). They vary in number from one to several and are usually located on the shins, though uncommonly they may occur on the trunk, arms

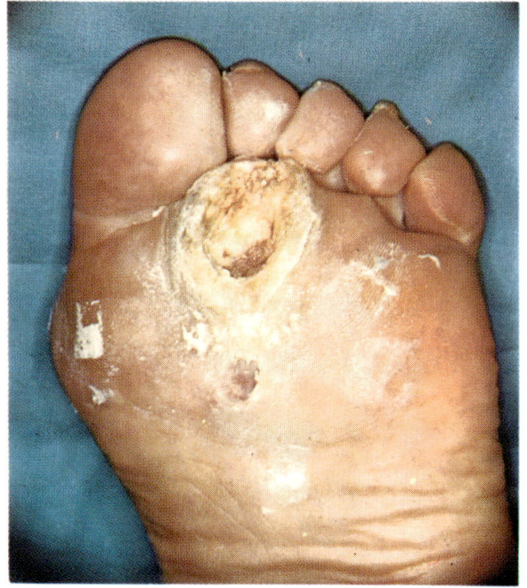

Fig. 4-1. Mal perforans in a diabetic can be especially serious; absence of pain sensation leads to neglect, carelessness, infection.

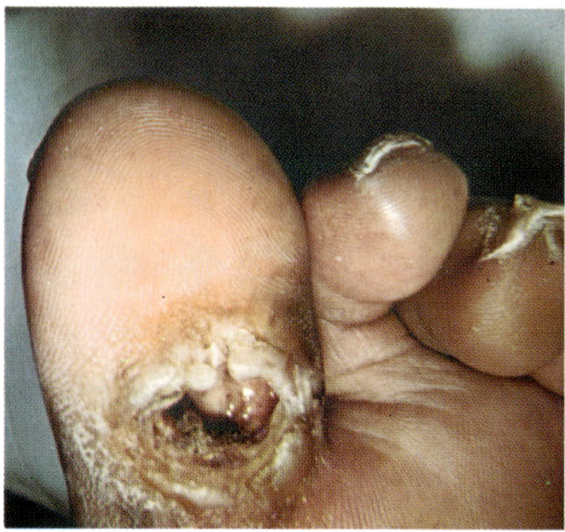

Fig. 4-2. Mal perforans. Appearance of ulcer following removal of crust.

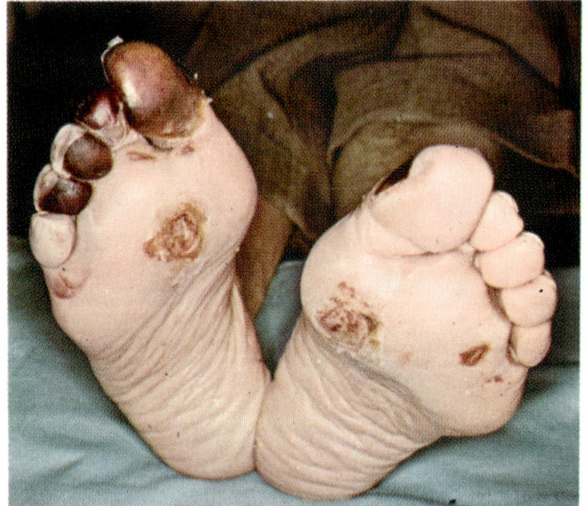

Fig. 4-3. Diabetic gangrene following application of hot water bottle in uncontrolled diabetic.

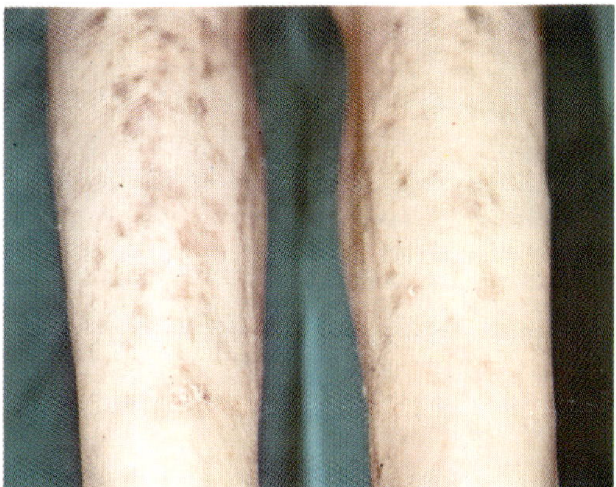

Fig. 4-4. Diabetic dermopathy. The lesions are discrete atrophic pigmented macules.

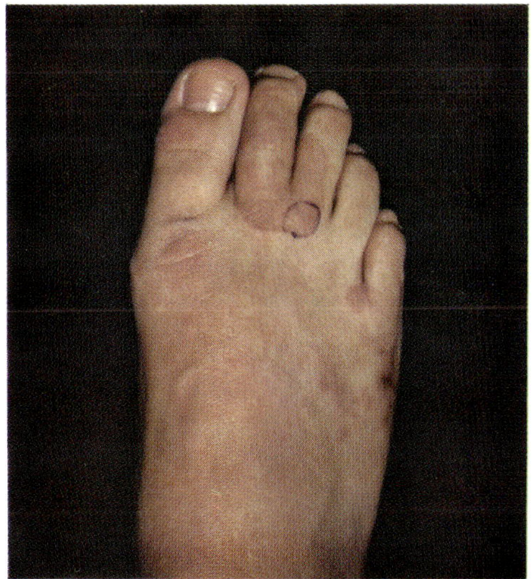

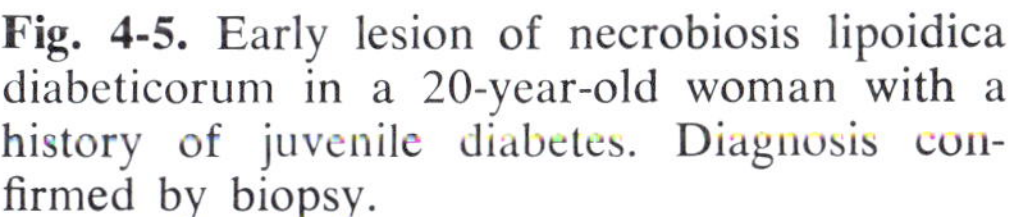

Fig. 4-5. Early lesion of necrobiosis lipoidica diabeticorum in a 20-year-old woman with a history of juvenile diabetes. Diagnosis confirmed by biopsy.

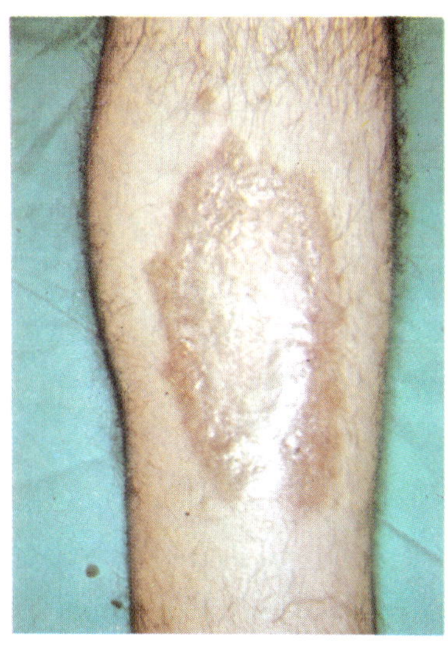

Fig. 4-6. Necrobiosis lipoidica diabeticorum. The atrophic, yellowish depressed lesion is characteristic.

or face. Patients of any age may be affected, but the majority occur in adults, women more often than men.

NLD usually is asymptomatic, though some itching may occur. In most instances the lesions are primarily a cosmetic problem but approximately one-third do develop ulcers within the sclerotic atrophic plaques which can be painful and slow to heal.

Therapy is not particularly successful but steroids with occlusion can be beneficial. Some authors have reported improvement in about half the cases treated with intralesional steroid injections.

Carotenosis

Carotenosis is a harmless yellowish discoloration of the skin seen occasionally in diabetics. It is caused by the presence of excess amounts of the pigment, carotene, which is contained in such foods as carrots and squash. The discoloration is most striking on the palms and soles and over bony prominences. The precise mechanism responsible for the development of carotenemia is not known, but the condition is innocent and improves upon dietary reduction of carotenes.

Xanthoma Diabeticorum

A rare complication of diabetes, occurring in approximately 0.1 percent of diabetics, xanthoma diabeticorum, presents as crops of papules and nodules appearing rather acutely over the trunk, buttocks, elbows, knees, oral mucous membranes, palms and soles. The papules are usually yellowish but may be erythematous and may show a surrounding inflammatory halo, thereby simulating pustules. The lesions may be tender and pruritic. Hypertriglyceridemia is a characteristic finding. With regulation of the diabetes and reduction of the blood lipid levels, the lesions disappear usually leaving no residue, though rarely some atrophy and pigmentation occur.

Idiopathic Bullae in Diabetics

Asymptomatic bullae, occurring without trauma on the dorsal surfaces of the feet of diabetics, which healed slowly without scarring have been described.[8] The etiology is unknown and is not consistently associated with neuropathy.

Therapy of Leg Lesions Associated with Diabetes

It is of utmost importance that the diabetic patient care for his feet with never-ending concern. A decreased blood supply of the lower leg and foot is a common accompaniment of diabetes. This underlies the development of cutaneous complications. Cutaneous fungal and bacterial infections may quickly transform from minor annoyances to major, occasionally fatal, complications. Minor trauma, whether mechanical as from ill-fitting shoes, thermal as from hot water bottles or chemical as from the injudicious use of topical home remedies, can result in chronic ulcerations with great potential for secondary infection and cellulitis. In addition, infection may precipitate diabetic acidosis and coma in a previously well-controlled diabetic patient. Thus the importance of proper prophylactic foot care and correct therapeutic measures for specific problems cannot be overemphasized.

Prophylactic foot care consists of wearing correctly fitting shoes and absorbent cotton socks and using a bland, absorbent foot powder. Keeping the feet dry and ventilated will reduce the incidence of bacterial and fungal infections.

When a cutaneous infection occurs, the patient should immediately be put on bed rest. Appropriate bacterial cultures and antibiotic sensitivity studies should be done. If the involved area is oozing, compresses should be employed. Specific systemic and/or topical antibacterial or antifungal agents should be utilized to eradicate the infection.

When ulcerations occur, presumably related to trauma in an area of skin which has a compromised vascularity, the same basic therapeutic measures of bed rest and bacterial studies should be carried out. For ischemic ulcers the head of the bed should be raised. Often bland compresses (saline), bed rest and patience will result in healing of the ulcer. When debris is considerable, an enzymatic ointment could be used to clear the ulcer base and then should be discontinued, since these agents do not contribute to further healing. Hydrogen peroxide soaks followed by Gelfoam powder packing daily is often helpful in healing an ulcer. When necessary, skin grafts may be indicated. However, in our experience such attempts at grafting are often undertaken prematurely without an adequate trial of conservative medical therapy and at times without due consideration of the decreased vascular supply to the area.

It is, of course, vital that the diabetes be maintained under good control.

References

1. Fitzpatrick, T. B.: Dermatologic lesions and diseases associated with diabetes. *In* Williams, R. H.: Diabetes: With a Chapter on Hypoglycemia. pp. 623-641. New York, Paul B. Hoeber, 1960.

2. *Ibid.*

3. Melin, H.: An atrophic circumscribed skin lesion in the lower extremities of diabetics. Acta Med. Scand., 176, Suppl. 423, 1964.

4. Binkley, G.W.: Dermopathy in diabetes mellitus, transactions of the Cleveland Dermatological Society, September 1964. Arch. Derm., *92*:106, 1965.

5. Binkley, G. W.: Dermopathy in the diabetic syndrome. Arch. Derm., *92*:625, 1965.

6. Bauer, M. F. *et al.*: Pigmented pretibial patches. Arch. Derm., *93*: 282, 1966.

7. Muller, S. A., and Winkelmann, R. K.: Necrobiosis lipoidica diabeticorum: a clinical and pathological investigation of 171 cases. Arch. Derm., *93*: 272, 1966.

8. Cantwell, A. R., Jr., and Martz, W.: Idiopathic bullae in diabetics. Arch. Derm., *96*: 42, 1967.

PRETIBIAL MYXEDEMA AND ACROPACHY

Localized myxedema is characterized by focal accumulation of ground substance; it is most commonly limited to the pretibial region. In 1840, von Basedow[1] described the disorder in a woman with exophthalmic goiter. Since that time the association of thyrotoxicosis, exophthalmos, and pretibial myxedema has been well recognized. Within recent years the localized myxedema syndrome has been enlarged to include a fourth, related condition, acropachy.[2,3] This disorder is a hypertrophic osteoarthropathy most frequently manifested as clubbing of the toes and soft tissue swelling of the extremities. It develops only after the other signs of the syndrome have become established.

Pretibial myxedema occurs in about 3 percent of patients with toxic diffuse goiter.[4] In approximately 50 percent of patients the lesions appear during the active hyperthyroid state; in the remainder they develop following treatment for the hyperthyroidism. In either case, the onset is apparently always subsequent to the development of exophthalmos. The sexes are equally affected.

The characteristic lesions are firm, nonpitting, irregular swellings, nodules or plaques which may be flesh-colored or pink to yellow and waxy. The overlying epidermis is thin and stretched; the follicles are prominent, imparting a "pigskin" appearance. The lesions appear bilaterally on the pretibial areas (Fig. 4-7), but they may be seen on the dorsa of the feet, the thighs, and, rarely, the abdomen. They may extend about the legs forming shinguard-like, thick heavy masses of uneven contour.[5] The hair in these lesions is often increased in amount, coarse and dry.

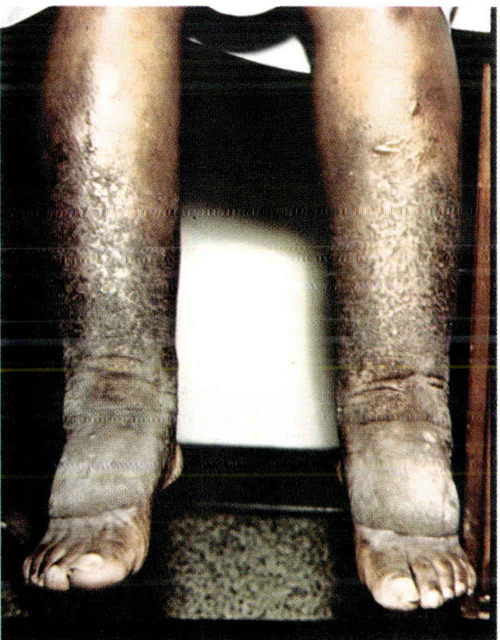

Fig. 4-7. Pretibial myxedema.

The changes evolve in a characteristic order (viz, hyperthyroidism, exophthalmos, pretibial myxedema, and acropachy). Acropachy occurs in less than 1 percent of patients with hyperthyroidism and always after therapy. Like the exophthalmos and pretibial myxedema, acropachy may run its course without obvious relationship to the level of thyroid function. It often continues to progress while the other manifestations of the syndrome persist unchanged or improve. Roentgenologic and histologic studies reveal increased vascularity and marked fibrosis associated with newly formed subperiosteal bone formation involving primarily the phalanges, metatarsals and metacarpals. Clubbing may or may not be seen in association with acropachy. It appears that clubbing is due to fibrosis and distended arteriovenous anastomoses lying between the nail and the phalanx.[6]

The histopathology of pretibial myxedema is characterized by the presence of large amounts of acid mucopolysaccharides, mainly hyaluronic acid, in the dermis, particularly the lower portion. There it occurs not only as individual threads and granules, but as extensive deposits causing wide separation of collagen bundles. In some areas there may be degeneration of collagen fibers, and in others there is new collagen formation with an increase in the number of fibroblasts. The latter are the source of hyaluronic acid.

The pathogenesis of pretibial myxedema has as yet not been definitively determined. Since the condition occurs in association with hyperthyroidism and exophthalmos, it was originally postulated that thyroid stimulating hormone (TSH) was mediating the disorder. Subsequent research into this problem has revealed that TSH is most likely not responsible since there is no correlation between TSH levels and hyperthyroidism and the presence or absence of exophthalmos or pretibial myxedema.[7]

Recent studies have shown that long-acting thyroid stimulator (LATS) is almost invariably elevated in patients with pretibial myxedema. LATS is quite distinct from TSH, and is not produced by the anterior pituitary, but from antibody-producing cells.[8] LATS is an abnormal gamma globulin which stimulates thyroid activity in an unusually long-acting fashion. It has been suggested that this globulin is involved in the production of the lesions, but as yet this is unproved.

Treatment

Local injection of triamcinolone suspension often produces resolution. In more widespread cases, fluorinated corticosteroid creams under occlusion often remarkably improve the condition. Local injection of hyaluronidase has no effect. Surgical excision is followed by recurrence in a few months.

References

1. Major, Ralph H.: Classic Descriptions of Disease. ed. 3, p. 283, Charles C. Thomas, Springfield, (Ill.) 1945.

2. Gimlette, T. M. D.: Thyroid acropachy. Lancet, *1*:22, Jan. 2, 1960.

3. Malkinson, F. D.: Hyperthyroidism, pretibial myxedema, and clubbing. Arch. Derm., *88*: 303, Sept., 1963.

4. Trotter, W.R., and Eden, K. C.: Localized pretibial myxedema in association with toxic goitre. Quart J. Med, *11*: 229, Oct., 1942.

5. Andrews, G. C., and Domonkos, A. N.: Diseases of the Skin. p. 145. Philadelphia, Saunders, 1963.

6. Lever, W. F.: Histopathology of the Skin. ed. 4, p. 429-432. Philadelphia, J. B. Lippincott, 1967.

7. Bluefarb, S.M., and Adams, L. A.: Hyperthyroidism, exophthalmos, pretibial myxedema, and early clubbing. Transactions of the Chicago Dermatological Society, May, 1966. Arch. Derm., *95*: 433, 1967.

8. Malkinson, F.D., and Furey, N.: Pretibial myxedema. Transactions of the Chicago Dermatological Society, Jan., 1967. Arch. Derm., *96*:737, 1967.

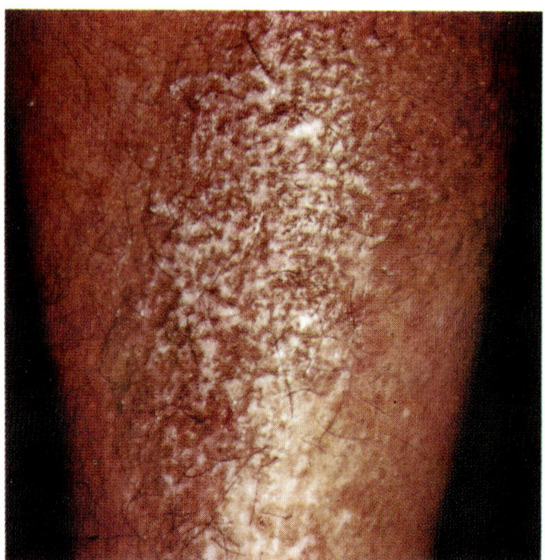

Fig. 4-8. Lichen amyloidosus. Patient's major complaint was intense pruritus.

LICHEN AMYLOIDOSUS

Lichen amyloidosus is a form of amyloidosis which is localized to the skin; the general health of the patient is not affected. The cause is unknown.

This local form of amyloidosis is characterized by an eruption of discrete, firm papules which vary in color from red to reddish-brown and occasionally are translucent. The papules may coalesce to form well-defined plaques. The eruption most frequently involves the lower extremities (Fig. 4-8) but may occur on the forearms, thighs and back. Pruritus is usually a prominent symptom, and because of the clinical appearance of the lesions and associated pruritus, lichen amyloidosus must be differentiated from lichen planus and lichen simplex chronicus. The diagnosis is established by histological and histochemical studies. The lesions of lichen amyloidosus tend to persist indefinitely.

The major constituent of amyloid deposits is a fibrous glycoprotein with a unique ultrastructure, chemical composition, and crystallographic pattern.[1] The amyloid substance in lichen amyloidosus has been shown to have the same characteristics as the amyloid in other forms of amyloidosis. Staining reactions are essentially those of acid or neutral mucopolysaccharides which comprise 1.5 percent of amyloid material. In sections stained with hematoxylin and eosin, the material is observed to be an amorphous pink substance. Histochemically,[2] amyloid demonstrates metachromasia with crystal violet and methyl violet stains. The substance stains red with Congo red and stains with PAS, alcian blue and Hale stains. These reactions are positive in frozen sections but may be negative in paraffin embedded sections. In routine sections amyloid can be demonstrated by staining with the Thioflavine-T stain because amyloid develops a fluorescence which can be observed when examined with a fluorescent microscope.

In the histopathology, deposits of amyloid are noted in the papillary bodies where they appear as homogenous masses which frequently contain clefts as a result of shrinkage during the processing of the material.

Treatment

Topical steroids under occlusion or local steroid infiltration has been helpful.

References

1. Cohen, A. S.: Pathogenesis of amyloidosis. Ann. Int. Med. (Editorial), *70*:418, Feb., 1969.

2. Hashimoto, K., Gross, B. G., and Lever, W. F.: Lichen amyloidosus - histochemical and electron microscopic studies. J. Invest. Derm., *45*: 204, 1965.

5

Eczematous Dermatitides

CONTACT DERMATITIS

Eczematous dermatitides account for a large proportion of skin diseases. The term, eczematous dermatitis, describes a morphologic-histologic picture; a qualifying adjective, for example, eczematous contact dermatitis includes an etiologic definition. Contact dermatitis is the most frequent type of eczematous dermatitis and is commonly observed on the lower extremities, especially the feet.

One has only to see the limping patient with oozing and painful eczematous contact dermatitis of the feet to know the serious nature of this disease. Not only is he susceptible to severe cellulitis, thrombophlebitis or lymphangitis, but often he is totally unable to carry on important daily activities. The well-trained physician can recognize the problem and successfully treat it. More important, he can discover the cause of the problem and prevent recurrence. The importance of a good history regarding onset, topical medications, types of shoes, and occupational and environmental factors cannot be overstressed.

Contact dermatitis is an inflammatory condition of the skin caused by external agents. Etiologically, it can be divided into primary irritant (toxic) and allergic contact dermatitis. The acute phase is characterized by erythema, edema, papulation, vesiculation, oozing, scaling and is accompanied by pruritus; chronic reactions show scaling, thickening, fissuring, lichenification and pigmentary changes. Histologically, acute contact dermatitis shows spongiosis, intra-epidermal vesiculation, and infiltration of inflammatory cells with vascular dilation in the upper dermis. Distinction between allergic and primary irritant reactions by clinical findings is often difficult; histological examination within several hours of the start of the dermatitis, as at patch test sites, is more informative. Allergic reactions show early perivascular accumulation of lymphocytes in the upper dermis; in irritant reactions, neutrophiles predominate. Chronic contact dermatitis appears as acanthosis, hyperkeratosis with areas of parakeratosis, and a predominantly lymphocytic infiltrate in the upper dermis.

A primary irritant is a substance that is always capable of causing tissue damage when applied for sufficient time and in sufficient concentration. A contact allergen is a substance that causes a hypersensitivity reaction. Characteristically, there is an induction period between an initial sensitizing exposure and development of the capacity to react to a subsequent exposure. With most allergens only a fraction of the population will develop contact allergy. In the irritant type, the chief variable is the substance itself; an antibody is not required (nonimmunological mechanism). In sensitization, the chief variable is the host; the intervention of an antibody is required (immunological mechanism).

The hypersensitivity is of the delayed type. Certain prerequisites must be satisfied to induce contact allergy: (1) surface contact, (2) penetration into the skin, (3) conjugation with a protein to form the antigen. Circulating antibodies have not been found. Like tuberculin sensitivity, contact allergy is mediated by lymphoid cells. Lymphocytes can transfer the sensitization to normal subjects.

The feet must resist the onslaught of many irritants and sensitizers under markedly adverse conditions. The feet are not often involved in irritant contact dermatitis in civilian life, but in the services where the military must spend many hours in wet footwear it is frequently seen. Among civilians, it occurs in those engaged in wet work where the feet are improperly protected and when footwear become soaked with water and degreasing agents. Kitchen workers may spill juices, dishwater and chemicals on their feet; mechanics may spill greases and oils.

On the other hand, the feet are common sites of allergic eczematous contact dermatitis. Frequently, the condition is misdiagnosed as tinea or "sweaty sock" dermatitis or remains unrecognized. A variety of factors play a role in the allergic type. The occlusive state produced by stockings and shoes inhibits the evaporation of moisture and results in increased water content of the stratum corneum. This promotes percutaneous absorption by as much as 100 times.[1] Hyperhidrosis can act as a precipitating factor. Sweating of the soles is under psychic influence and can be markedly increased in times of emotional stress.[2] Sweat also has the capacity to leach out chemicals, such as chromium salts, from shoes.[3] Alkaline solutions damage the horny layer by breaking cross-links in keratin and thereby allowing penetration of water with subsequent swelling. Inflammatory changes in the epidermis, whether caused by irritants, sensitizers or simple friction, further facilitate percutaneous absorption of noxious materials. Scratches and frankly denuded areas caused by friction permit unrestricted penetration.

On the feet, contact allergy is commonly caused by four major groups of materials: wearing apparel, components of shoes and stockings; applied medicaments; appliances used on feet; and substances encountered in certain occupational exposures. In particular, shoe allergens have evoked much enthusiasm for investigation among dermatologists.

SHOE DERMATITIS

History

Contact dermatitis from shoes is a problem that must surely date back to the first days that man strapped chemically treated materials to his feet. Yet, it was not until 1929 that Bloch first documented a case of dermatitis of the feet caused by sensitivity to shoe leather.[4] Subsequent reports were quick to follow. In 1949, Gaul and Underwood[5] called attention to the fact that many dermatoses of the feet are misdiagnosed as fungal infections and are in reality caused by irritants and allergens.

In 1952, Blank and Miller[6] tested 24 cases of shoe dermatitis with 10 representative antioxidants and 17 accelerators. They determined that the most common offenders were the rubber additives monobenzyl ether of hydroquinone, 2-mercaptobenzothiazole and tetramethylthiuram monosulfide. Rubber additives were further emphasized by Shatin and Reisch[7] in 1954. In the 1950's and 1960's several studies showed the importance of the tanning agents in leather as a cause of dermatitis.[8,9,10]

Incidence

The number of cases of contact dermatitis varies with climate and with the particular compounds used in preparing shoes. Shatin and Reisch[11] reported that 1 in 10 cases hospitalized at a V. A. hospital in New York City because of dermatitis of the feet was diagnosed as shoe dermatitis. This was 2 percent of the total dermatologic admissions to that hospital over a 5-year period. In a study of 213 patients with shoe dermatitis over a 13-year period in England,[12,13] the ages ranged from 3 to 80 years, with about 85 percent between 12 and 60 years. There were 3 times as many women as men. It has been speculated that the changing styles, colors, and materials in women's shoes allow women to be exposed to many different sensitizers.[14] Also, the fashion of not wearing hose allows more intimate contact of shoe to skin.

Structure of Shoes

The basic structure of all men's shoes is fairly similar regardless of style or trademark.[15] This also applies to the oxford worn by women and children. In brief, the sole usually consists of an innersole of leather, a midsole of fabric or reclaimed rubber and an outersole of leather, plastic or rubber. The upper portion consists of outside leather, waterproofed paper, the box toe and the lining. Adhesives are used throughout.

The box toe is one of three general types: rubber, thermoplastic, celastic. Linings may be dyed and may be impregnated with fungicides to prevent mildew. Women's dress shoes are of lighter construction and contain fewer materials. Often the upper portion consists of several straps of leather or fabric lined with leather. The sole may consist of several sheets of leather only. Moccasins have neither a box toe nor a lining.

Diagnosis

The diagnosis of allergic contact dermatitis depends upon history, an eczematous eruption and its localization. Special testing (patch test) is valuable in defining the causal agent.

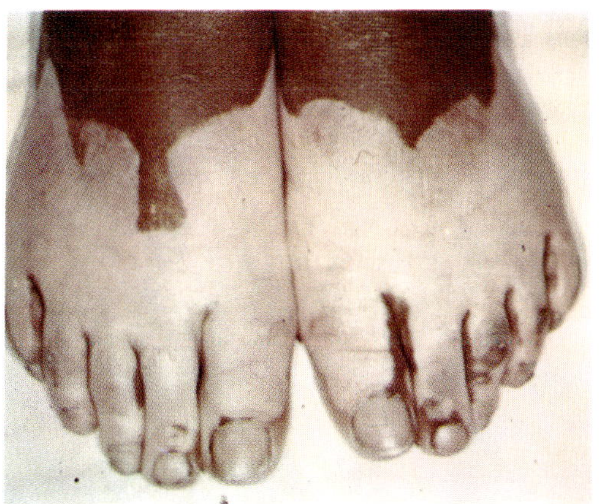

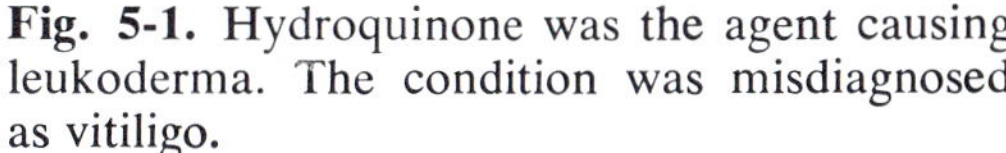

Fig. 5-1. Hydroquinone was the agent causing leukoderma. The condition was misdiagnosed as vitiligo.

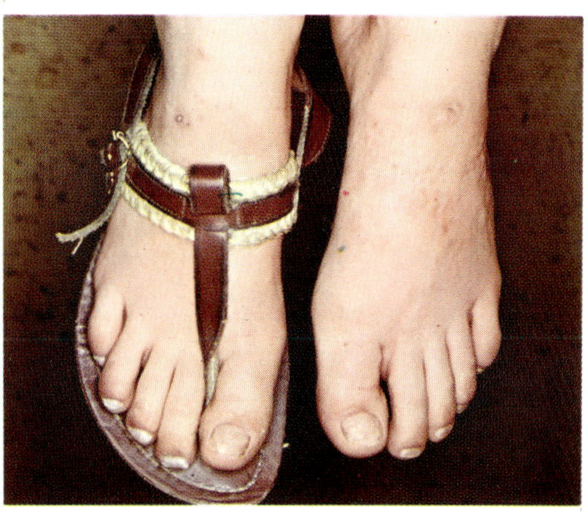

Fig. 5-2. Characteristic distribution of contact dermatitis in patient wearing thong sandals.

A good history is essential. Time relationship of wearing a new pair of shoes to onset of the dermatitis is important. However, in many cases of bona fide shoe dermatitis there may be no such history. Also, some patients known to be sensitive are able to wear shoes containing the offending agent successfully for months before developing a dermatitis. Often, a recurrence of the dermatitis occurs in hot weather when there is excessive sweating of the feet.

Clinical Picture. In the classic case, shoe dermatitis presents as an eczematous dermatitis beginning on the dorsal aspect of the big toe with eventual extension to other toes, sparing the toe webs and soles. In those cases where hydroquinone is the sensitizing agent, the presenting lesions at these sites may be patches of leucoderma (Fig. 5-1) without features of eczematization. It is reasonable to suspect this area as the common site of involvement, because dorsal skin is thinner and contains numerous follicular openings through which materials can penetrate, and because more intimate contact of sensitizers with the dorsum of the toes often follows excessive friction and wearing away of the inner shoe linings of the box toe. The majority of cases reported by various investigators[16,17,18] had dorsal surface involvement. The soles are another common site of involvement. In a series of cases reported by Cronin,[19] the soles were involved in 59 out of 77 patients and were the only affected sites in 28 of these patients; the dorsal toe surfaces, however, were the predominant areas of involvement.

The type of shoe alters the distribution of the dermatitis. Unusual patterns can result; for instance thong sandals, many styles of which consist of only a single thong between one or more toes and a strap or two across the instep or heel, has caused a dermatitis pattern which matches the areas contacted by the straps (Fig. 5-2).

At times, during acute exacerbations of shoe dermatitis, the patient may present "id-like" lesions on the hands or even widespread or generalized eruptions, especially following overtreatment or secondary infections. One may speculate that these distant flares represent the hematogenous dissemination of bacterial products from superimposed infections or of fungal products from dormant sites of tinea, or of altered keratin from the affected sites, or from drugs used topically which have the capacity to be absorbed percutaneously and so act as drug allergens.

Causative Agents. Components of shoes.

Rubber and Rubber Adhesives. The rubber in shoes today is made either from

1. Natural rubber: latex, an emulsion of isoprene in an aqueous phase;
2. Synthetic rubber: polyisoprene and butadiene polymers;
3. A combination of both natural and synthetic rubber.

Rubber appears in the soles, in the box toe and in rubber adhesives; it contains accelerators and antioxidants to make it more serviceable. The rubber additives present in the soles are usually responsible for contact dermatitis at these areas. The rubber box toe is one of the commonest causes of shoe dermatitis, the actual sensitizers being the rubber adhesives used to glue the lining to the upper leather. These are usually the rubber accelerators such as 2-mercaptobenzothiazole or tetramethylthiuram monosulfide, or antioxidants such as monobenzyl ether of hydroquinone.[20] The rubber box toe is popular because it is inexpensive.

Recently, adhesives and cements also have been examined for allergens. Adhesives contain: rubber with antioxidants and accelerators; ether as the volatile phase; plasticizers, phthalic esters that improve plasticity of rubber and facilitate vulcanization, and phenolic resins. Brandao[21] reported that all of his 16 shoe dermatitis patients were sensitive to dilute solutions of phenolic resins supplied by shoe manufacturers. A high incidence of hypersensitivity to phenolic resins has been documented by other investigators.[22,23] Suurmond and Mijnssen[24] in the Netherlands found that 8 out of 15 patients were positive to phenolic resins and 6 out of 15 patients were positive to accelerators and antioxidants.

The celastic box toe is composed of cotton flannel impregnated with pyroxylin, a cellulose nitrate and includes in addition an inorganic fire retardant, a mold retardant and a special solvent. The special solvent cements the lining and leather completely, negating the use of rubber cement. The celastic box toe is generally considered dermatologically harmless.[25]

The thermoplastic toe is a third form consisting of polystyrene, polyvinyl acetate or acrylic resins. They are rarely sensitizers. Shoes made with polystyrene toe boxes, however, contain butadiene which is a synthetic rubber.

Tanning Agents. The many compounds used in various steps of the tanning procedure have been tabulated by Brandao.[26] In his series, chromates, vegetable tannins, and aldehydes are the principal materials.

There has been much controversy as to whether the hexavalent or the trivalent chromium is more significant in shoe dermatitis. The trivalent species is used to tan leather and is theoretically in close chemical combination with the hide protein. We have demonstrated that trivalent chromium is extractable from chrome-tanned leathers by human sweat. We have also shown that hexavalent chromium is present as well[27] and it is this form, because of its higher sensitizing potential, that is generally considered to be the more likely offender.[28]

The incidence of shoe dermatitis to chromium compounds varies. Scutt[29] reported that of 67 naval ratings who returned from the tropics with dermatitis of the dorsa of the feet, 45 reacted to 0.25 percent potassium dichromate. Fisher[30] found that 20 percent of his cases of shoe dermatitis were caused by allergic reactions to the dichromates. Bett,[31] on the other hand, found that dichromates play a rather minor role. Samitz and Gross[32] reported that of 28 workers with known sensitivity to dichromate, only one developed a shoe dermatitis and in this case sensitivity to rubber materials in his shoes was not tested. Also, in Cronin's series of 213 cases[33] of shoe dermatitis, only 12 cases were positive to 0.5 percent potassium dichromate and 3 of 13 cases tested were positive to 10 percent basic chromic sulfate.

Vegetable tanning is generally used for processing hides to make heavy leathers. In the past, vegetable tannins have not been considered to cause dermatitis.[34,35] Recently, however, Cronin[36] has shown that all of 12 patients tested with semichrome leather (containing vegetable tans) and East Indian vegetable-tanned leathers were consistently positive. We also have observed a similar finding in an outbreak of shoe dermatitis from a leather sandal imported from India. Cronin has determined that vegetable tans are in fact complex mixtures of chemicals, mainly polyphenolic substances of the pyrogallol and catechol type. In Cronin's opinion, it is vegetable-tanned rather than chrome-tanned leather which is now the most common cause of shoe dermatitis in England. This is an interesting new finding and emphasizes the need for up-to-date testing and analysis of ever-changing shoe materials.

Aldehyde tanning, as with formaldehyde, is used in white skins such as "white kids" or "bucks." A positive patch test reaction to formaldehyde in a patient with foot dermatitis is therefore significant.

Dyes. Leather dyeing is done principally with the "azoaniline" group of dyes and so well fixed to the leather in the manufacturing process that shoe dye dermatitis is extremely rare.[37] Suurmond and Mijnssen[38] reported a series of 15 patients with 3 positive to paraphenylenediamine; however, all 3 had positive reactions to other shoe materials as well. It is important to note that dyes can be more easily leached from fabric and plastic shoes and from redyed shoes than from leather. In these instances dyes must be recognized as likely contactants.

Miscellaneous Substances. Other contactants in shoes are rare causes of dermatitis: antimildew agents, such as mercaptobenzothiazole, paranitrophenol, salicylanilide and inorganic mercury compounds; nickel present in eyelets, buckles, ornaments and arch supports.

Footgear other than regular shoes can also be offenders. Vinyl and unpolymerized acrylic resins, formaldehyde, antioxidants and plasticizers used in plastic shoes can all be allergenic. Rubber overshoes, especially galoshes, bathing shoes, sneakers, special shoes used in various athletic activities and bedroom slippers may be responsible for allergic contact dermatitis on the feet.

A new urethane material called Corfam is currently a popular replacement for leather; to date, no instance of Corfam sensitivity has been reported.

STOCKING DERMATITIS

Stocking dermatitis is often related to the dyes or to the detergents used in laundering. Although dermatitis from nylon stockings has been reported, most cases are actually caused by sensitivity to azo dyes which may cross-react with paraphenylenediamine and related rubber chemicals.[39]

In stocking dermatitis, the shape of the stocking may be outlined on the leg (Fig. 5-3). Typical sites of involvement, however, are the feet,

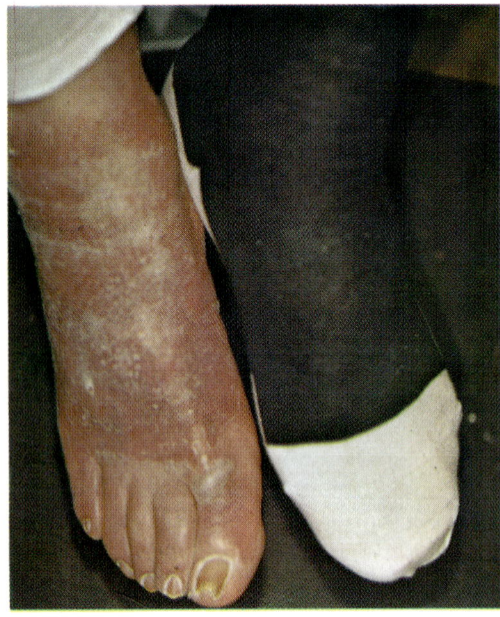

Fig. 5-3. Contact dermatitis due to stocking dye.

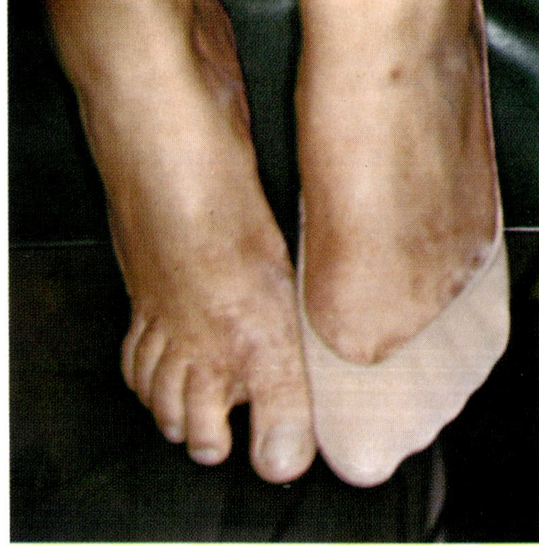

Fig. 5-4. Note interesting distribution of the eruption which follows the elastic band in the Peds. The sensitizing agent was 2-mercaptobenzothiazole.

popliteal fossae and inner thighs. In a few instances, with localization to the feet, the eruption can be mistaken for shoe dermatitis, but is probably due to sweat and friction inside the shoe, especially on the anterior part of the foot. Slight involvement in other areas such as the popliteal fossae and inner thighs is a valuable clue but is usually overlooked by the patient. Patch testing with the stocking confirms the diagnosis.

Peds, frequently worn by women who go without stockings, may cause contact dermatitis. We have observed rubber sensitivity from the elastic band which encircles the ped. The eruption is confined to a moccasin pattern (Fig. 5-4).

Von H. Suter[40] described 11 cases of dermatitis to polyamide stockings. Without exception, dyes were incriminated and no case of sensitization was caused by polyamide itself, by substances used in the preparation of fibers, or by antistatic materials.

The use of elastic stockings has also been responsible for contact dermatitis in patients allergic to rubber. The eruption in these patients conforms to areas covered by the special stockings. Also included under this category is contact dermatitis caused by garters. Rubber again is the sensitizer, the eruption being localized to sites covered by the garters.

Gibson[41] describes a "sweaty sock dermatitis" due to occlusive footwear that, unlike contact dermatitis, involves the web areas. This dermatitis is due to maceration by sweat and is seen in children whose feet perspire excessively and who wear either stockings of synthetic fibers or sneakers for prolonged periods.

MEDICATION DERMATITIS

One of the leading causes of dermatological disease is overtreatment. With our preoccupation with health and the influence of television and other advertising media, feet are constantly inundated with a host of creams, lotions, powders and ointments. We suffer from a plethora of absorbents, analgesics, antiseptics, anti-inflammatory, antibacterial and antifungal agents and keratolytics to be applied, supposedly for our comfort.

Almost any medicament, proprietary or prescribed, applied to normal or damaged skin will sensitize some persons (Fig. 5-5), although

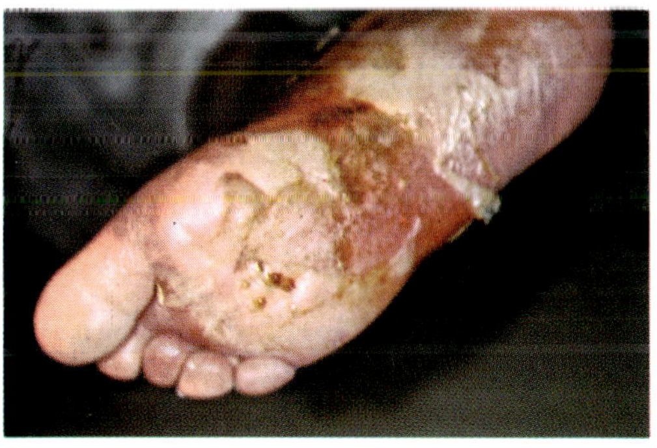

Fig. 5-5. Contact dermatitis caused by spray used to treat "tired feet." Patch tests were positive for formaldehyde and menthol, constituents of the spray.

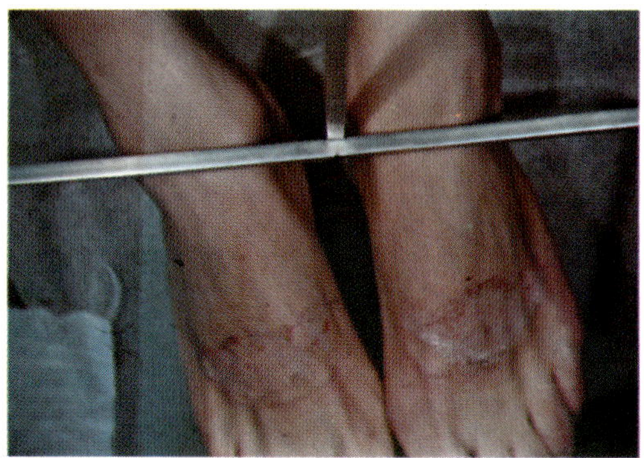

Fig. 5-6. The contact dermatitis conforms to the metal buckle on the shoe. Patient showed positive reaction to nickel on patch test.

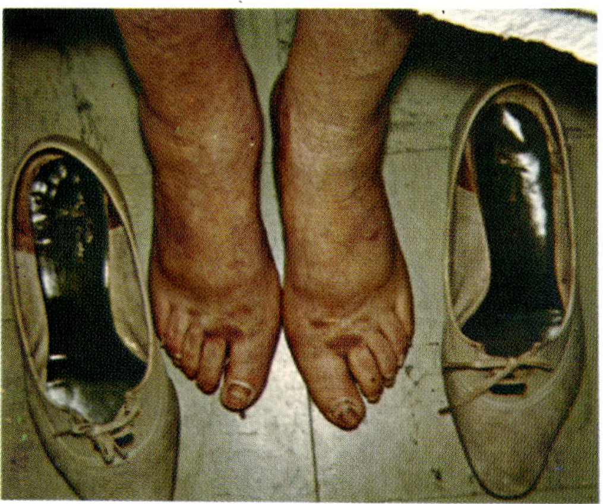

Fig. 5-7. Allergic contact photodermatitis. Note line of demarcation where shoes have covered toes.

weak sensitizers rarely do so unless used on burns or severe dermatitis.[42] Neomycin and topical formulations containing sensitizing preservatives[43,44] may play a significant role in contact dermatitis. Patch testing of components in recommended concentrations should be carried out. Often a trial application of a suspected allergen to a small limited test area will be helpful.

APPLIANCES USED ON FEET

Included under this group are arch supports, orthopedic braces, elastic supports, athletic tape, pads and other devices used to relieve painful foot problems. Nickel, rubber compounds and plastics are the offenders (Fig. 5-6).

OCCUPATIONAL DERMATITIS

In many industries, the feet of workers are exposed to a variety of chemicals which have the capacity to sensitize the skin. Contact with these agents usually results from working in bare feet, and from leakage of solutions spilling over the shoes and feet. An example of the latter is the herbicide dermatitis of farmers, reported by Spencer.[45] Another type of exposure may be due to components of specially designed work shoes and rubber boots worn in various occupations. The vagaries of rubber boot dermatitis in fishermen were described by Ross.[46]

MISCELLANEOUS CONTACT DERMATITIS

An unusual dermatitis of the feet is the allergic contact photodermatitis, resulting from contact with photosensitizing fungicides used to treat athlete's foot. In some patients with a long-standing allergic

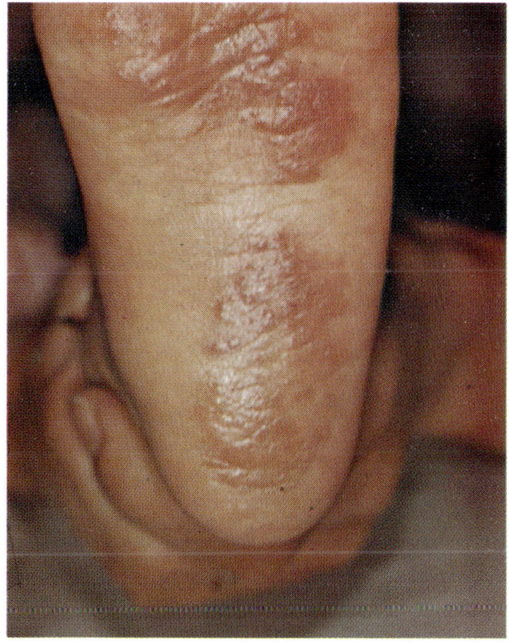

Fig. 5-8. Contact dermatitis due to components of inner sole.

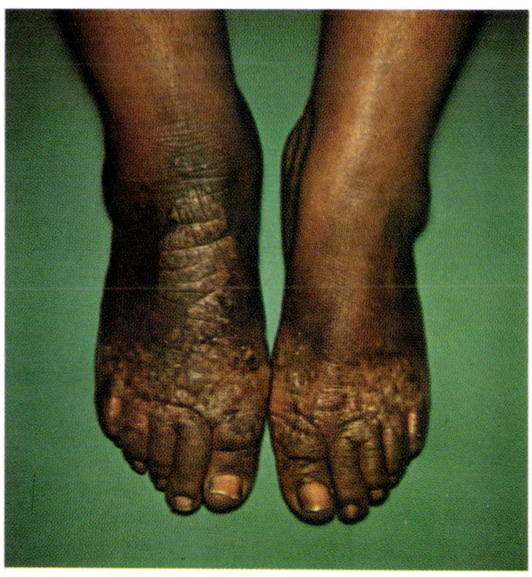

Fig. 5-10. Chronic shoe dermatitis. The lichenified lesions had been treated as a neurodermatitis.

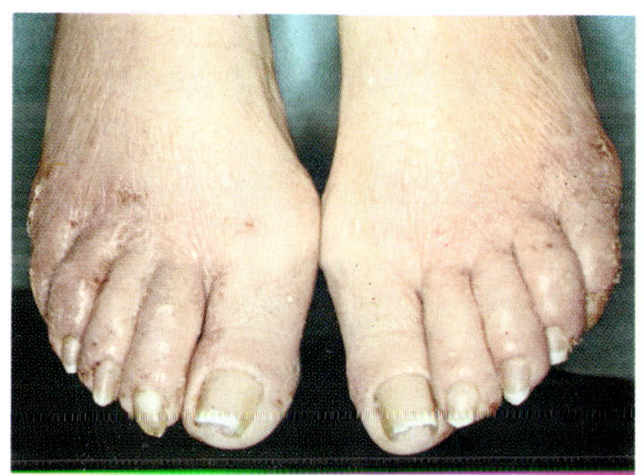

Fig. 5-9. Shoe dermatitis from box toe. Rubber adhesives used to glue the lining were sensitizers.

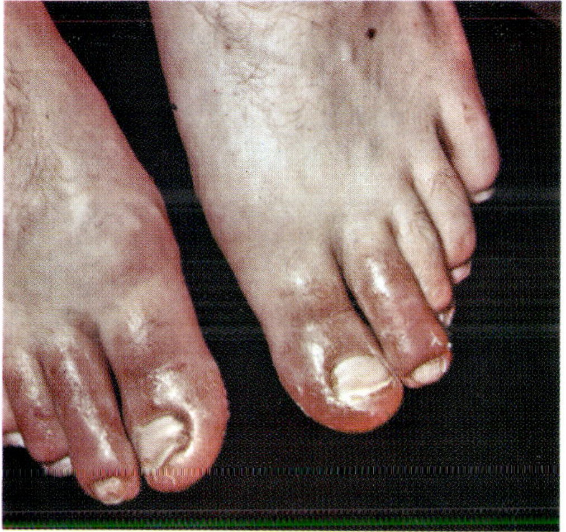

Fig. 5-11. A classical picture of box toe dermatitis. The sensitizer was tetramethylthiuram monosulfide.

contact photodermatitis, hyperpigmentation and lichenification have been so striking that the affected areas resemble a chronic neurodermatitis (Fig. 5-7).*

*See also illustrations on pp. 121-123, Fig. 5-8, Fig. 5-9, Fig. 5-10, Fig. 5-11, Fig. 5-12, Fig. 5-13, Fig. 5-14, Fig. 5-15, Fig. 5-16, and Fig. 5-17.

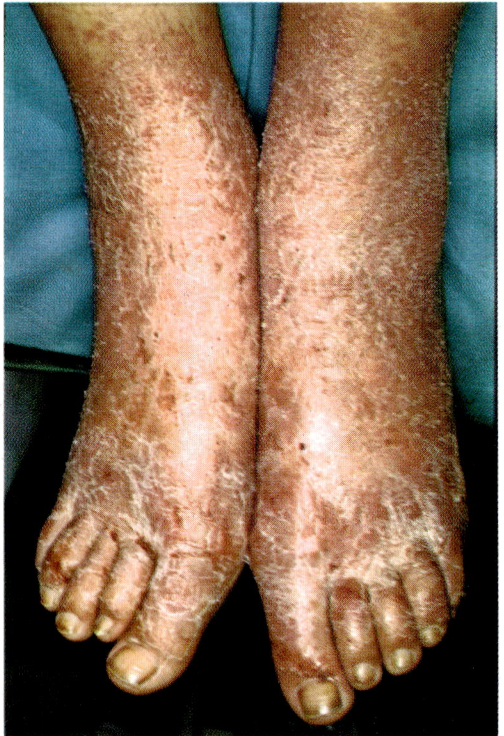

Fig. 5-12. This patient could not wear shoes and was almost completely incapacitated. She had been treated for neurodermatitis for 4 years.

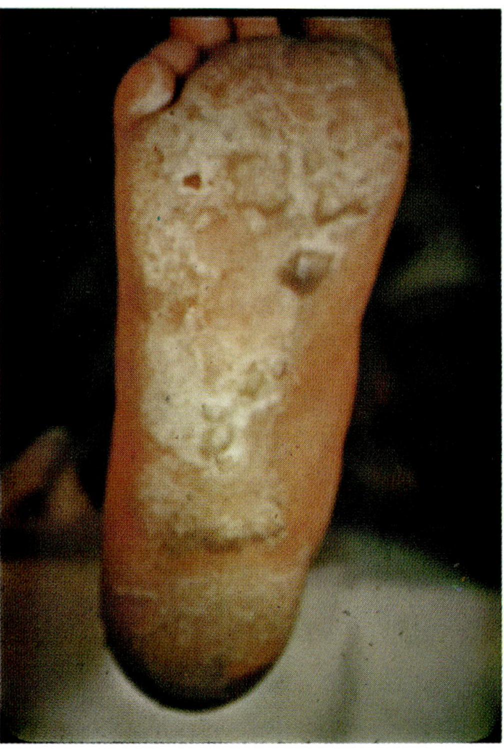

Fig. 5-14. Contact dermatitis from rubber additives in glue used in soles. The sensitizer was 2-mercaptobenzothiazole.

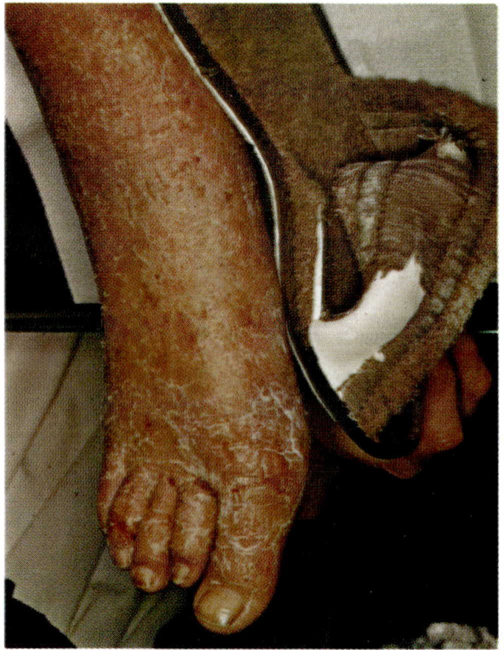

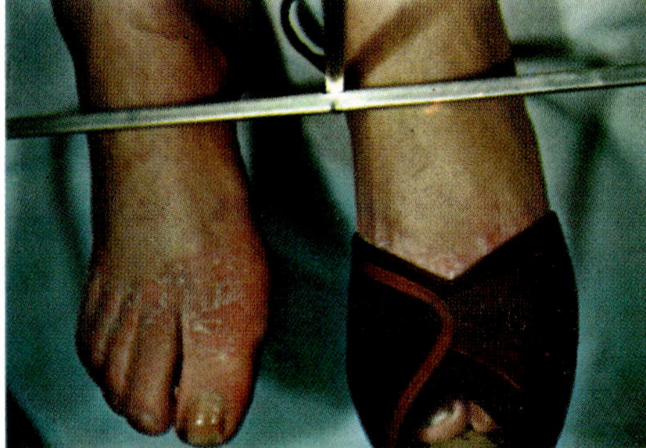

Fig. 5-15. Contact dermatitis from lining in the uppers of the shoe.

Fig. 5-13. The same patient (Fig. 5-12) could get around only in soft bedroom slippers. When the bedroom slippers were stripped, foam rubber was exposed. Patch tests confirmed a rubber sensitivity.

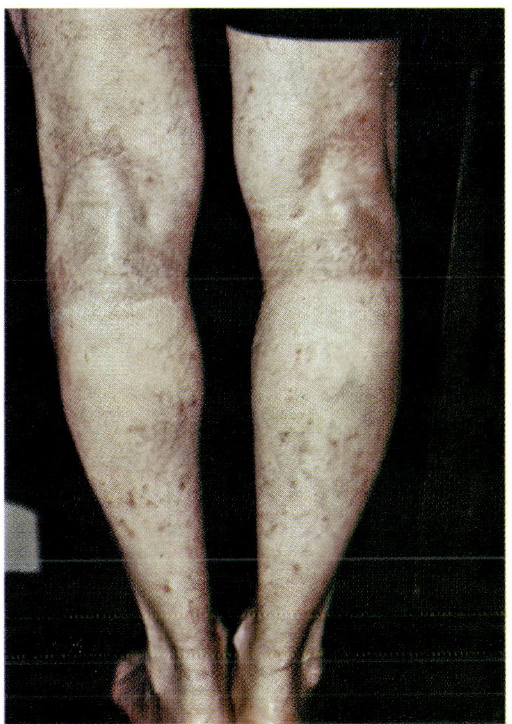

Fig. 5-16. The rubber in garters was responsible for contact dermatitis on upper legs.

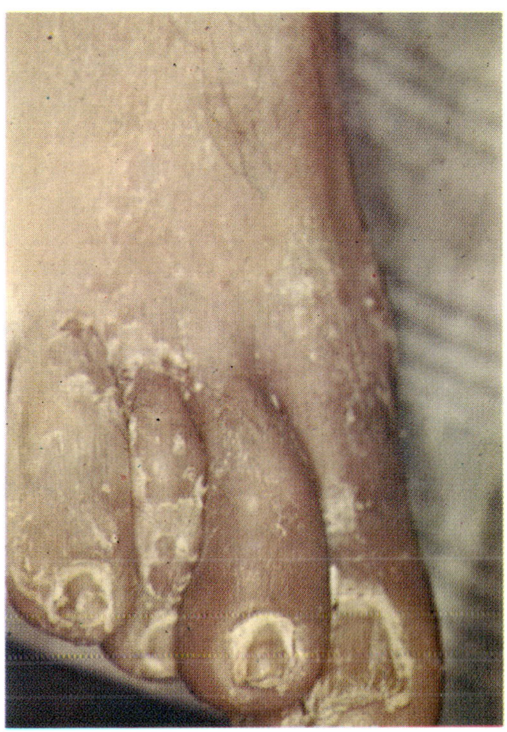

Fig. 5-17. Box-toe dermatitis with superimposed pyocyaneous infection.

Patch Tests

Allergic eczematous contact dermatitis on the feet may be so characteristic that it is readily recognized from history and examination. Clinical acumen and a high index of suspicion are the physician's greatest tools in diagnosing shoe dermatitis. Often, the only convincing evidence for a shoe dermatitis is the disappearance of a rash after substituting shoes with a totally different construction (e.g., plastic or cloth instead of leather shoes).

The patch test is the means of establishing the cause of contact dermatitis. It is a specific procedure which reproduces the patient's clinical disease in miniature and is used solely in allergic contact dermatitis and not at all in irritant dermatitis. Although patch testing may seem a simple procedure, the manner of application and the interpretation of the tests require the experience of the expert.

The test material is applied directly to the normal skin on a small square (0.5 sq. cm.) of white cotton cloth. The patch is covered by a larger piece of cellophane and both kept in place by a piece of adhesive. Commercial patches are available and simple to use. The material remains on the skin for 48 hours to promote penetration and allow time for the delayed reaction to develop. The upper part of the back is the preferable patch test site. The patient is instructed to remove the test material at any time from any site of burning or pain. Readings are made 30 minutes after removal of the patches and the sites are reexamined after 2 to 5 days for delayed reactions (Figs. 5-18, 5-19). Often, however, the patch test is unreliable because (1) the testing conditions do not duplicate the adverse conditions of the feet in shoes, and (2) testing materials may not include the proper allergens.

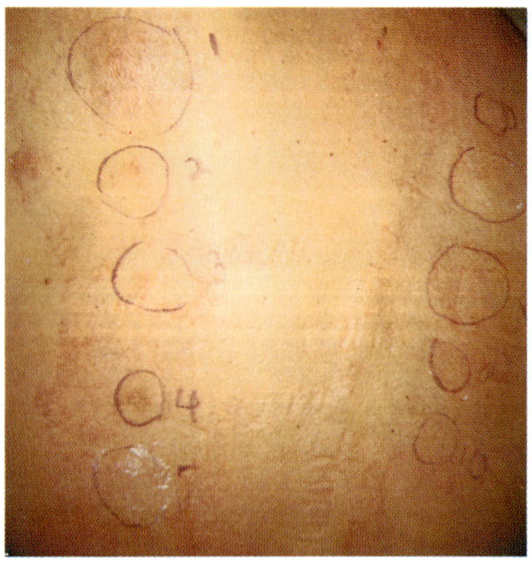

Fig. 5-18. Positive patch tests to tetramethylthiuram (patient, Fig. 5-11).

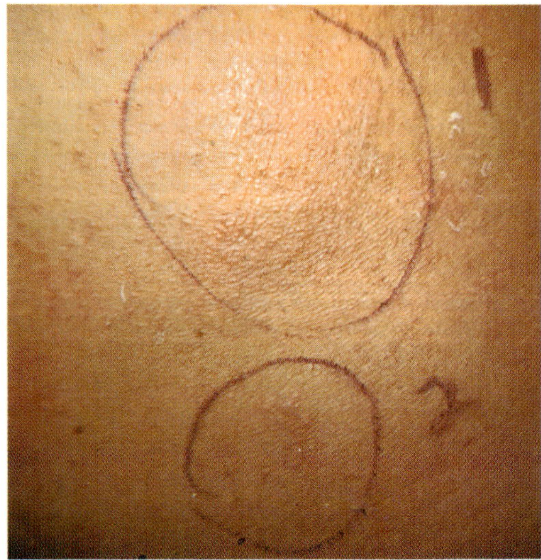

Fig. 5-19. Close-up of positive patch test (patient, Fig. 5-11).

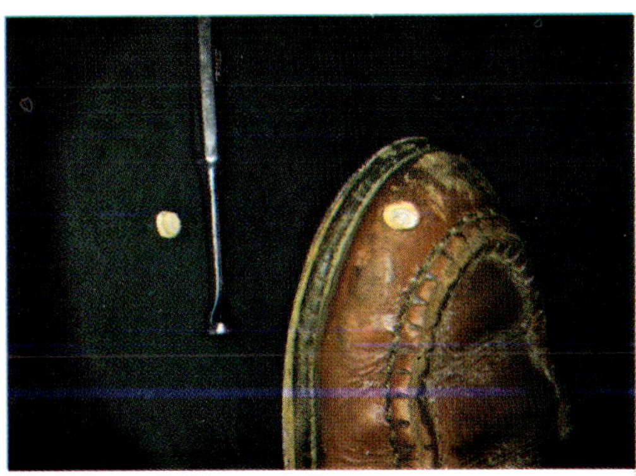

Fig. 5-20. A skin biopsy punch is used to remove leather and lining for patch testing.

A shoe "screening tray" is a useful adjunct for patch testing. Fisher has recommended a list of standard substances; however, revisions are needed every few years because new products are always being introduced.

Diagnostic Series for Allergic Shoe Dermatitis*

1. Rubber box toe material (as is).
2. 1 percent monobenzylether of hydroquinone in petrolatum (rubber antioxidant).
3. 1 percent mercaptobenzothiazole in petrolatum (rubber accelerator).
4. 1 percent tetramethylthiuram monosulfide in petrolatum (rubber accelerator).
5. 1 percent hexamethylenetetramine in petrolatum (rubber accelerator).
6. 1 percent phenyl beta napthylamine in petrolatum (rubber antioxidant).
7. 0.25 percent potassium dichromate in aqueous solution (tanning agent).
8. 5 percent formaldehyde in aqueous solution (tanning agent for white shoes).
9. 2 percent paraphenylenediamine in petrolatum (may cross-react with shoe dyes).
10. 5 percent nickel sulfate in aqueous solution (eyelets, buckles, tips of shoelaces).

In our experience it is preferable to patch test patients with small pieces of the components of their own shoes. Specimens are obtained easily by using a 6 to 8 mm. skin biopsy punch (Fig. 5 20). This provides a satisfactory sample of all the shoe materials. The lining is separated from the leather and the actual materials are then applied "glue" surface facedown directly on the skin.

*Dr. A. A. Fisher (reference No. 17).

Treatment

The first principle in the treatment of allergic eczematous contact dermatitis is to identify and eliminate the sensitizer. Cure cannot be attained unless contact with the causal agent is avoided. Thus, it is of primary importance that the patient cease wearing the shoes or type of stocking to which he has shown a positive patch test, or to avoid contact with topical medicaments and occupational sensitizers.

Management of the individual case depends upon the stage of the eruption and the severity of the inflammatory reaction.

Local Measures. For the acute stage:

1. Local rest and elevation of the affected feet according to the severity and extent of the dermatitis.
2. Interdict use of soaps
3. Wet dressings such as Burow's solution (1:40 to 1:20) and saline solution are simple and effective. Compresses or soaks should be applied every 3 to 4 hours for 15 to 20 minutes. Clean sheeting, or muslin or a turkish towel are good dressing materials. Do not use plastic or other impervious material to prevent evaporation.

   BluBoro powder packets (Derm-Arts Laboratories), Buro-Sol (Doak Pharmacal Co., Inc.), Domeboro Tablets (Dome Laboratories) are convenient proprietaries for preparing Burow's solution.

   When the exudative or oozing phase subsides, the following may be used:
4. Simple pastes with Burow's solution applied as fixed dressings.

Burow's solution	1 part
Aquaphor	2 parts
Lassar's paste	3 parts

5. Corticosteroid creams. These anti-inflammatory agents can be applied following compressing or on the dry skin. We have found Kenalog 0.025 percent, Valisone 0.1 percent, Synalar 0.025 percent, and Cordran 0.025 percent creams effective agents in this stage. Topical antibiotics may be used when secondary infection is present. These are often combined in the steroid creams. Dressings should be light, comfortable and nonocclusive.

For the dry, scaly and thickened stages of eczematous eruptions, the following are suggested: ointments containing corticosteroids or creams and ointments containing tar or iodochlorhydroxyquin (Vioform). Corticosteroid creams may be used under a plastic film for short periods.

With ambulation, open shoes (sandals or shoes in which the box toes have been cut away) are recommended for short periods of time until complete involution of the eruption takes place.

Systemic Measures. Occasionally, secondary infection of cutaneous lesions may require oral or parenteral administration of antibiotics. Bacterial cultures and sensitivity tests to determine the antibiotic of choice are advisable and will afford a more direct attack on the infectious process.

Oral corticosteroids may be indicated in severe disabling cases. They should be used with caution and only by practitioners experienced in their use and aware of their adverse reactions and contraindications. When such treatment is necessary it should be for short-term use, usually 2 or 3 weeks. Initial high doses are tapered off gradually to prevent a "rebound" of the dermatitis. The following regimen is effective in most instances:

40 mg. prednisone or its equivalent (10 mg. q. i. d.) for 2 to 3 days,
30 mg. (10 mg. t. i. d.) for 2 days,
20 mg. (10 mg. b. i. d.) for 3 days,
15 mg. (5 mg. t. i. d.) for 3 days,
10 mg. (5 mg. b. i. d.) for 3 days,
5 mg. daily for 3 days

This can be modified by an initial intramuscular injection of a long-acting steroid suspension (Kenalog IM, Aristocort Forte, Celestone Soluspan) given on the first day followed by oral therapy with corticosteroids, as shown in the above schedule.

Following his recovery, it is essential that the patient be instructed in measures to help prevent recurrences. Measures to control hyperhidrosis are valuable. The causative agent, be it shoes, stockings, topical medicament or occupational exposure, must be avoided. The problem of stockings and topical medicaments is simple to correct. Finding shoes that are free of the particular sensitizer may be more difficult. Patients should be given explicit advice as to the type of shoes to be worn and the places to purchase them. Specific examples are unlined moccasins, shoes made with canvas, cloth and plastic uppers; shoes with celastic box toes for patients sensitive to rubber and its adhesives in rubber box toe shoes; vegetable-tanned shoes for those reacting to chrome-tanned shoes. Fisher[47] lists manufacturers and shops where such shoes can be bought in many metropolitan centers and Hack[48] provides the addresses of firms which manufacture special shoes and stockings. The Musebeck Shoe Company (Oconomowoc, Wisconsin 53066) manufactures shoes using vegetable-tanned leather and has eliminated all rubber cements in their shoes. The company is most cooperative in supplying the physician with samples of the materials used in their shoes for patch testing and a style folder which will give the patient an idea of the shoes available.

ATOPIC DERMATITIS

The term atopy was coined by Coca to describe a group of allergic diseases characterized by a strong hereditary background. The designation includes hay fever, asthma and atopic dermatitis. Reagins which have the capacity to be transferred to nonatopic individuals by the Prausnitz-Kustner (P-K) test prove the existence of circulating antibodies. In atopic dermatitis, however, it is difficult to assign the cause solely to an antigen-antibody reaction because the disease depends on the interplay of numerous constitutional and precipitating factors. As a rule, the value of skin testing in atopic dermatitis is slight, and treatment by specific desensitization is seldom helpful and at times may cause aggravation of the skin lesions.

Most characteristic of atopic dermatitis are its exacerbations and remissions. Factors in producing remissions may be changes in mode of life and season. Factors producing exacerbations may be heat, humidity and perspiration, exposure to certain antigens either by injection, inhalation or ingestion, infection, greasy topical medicaments, stress, overwork and fatigue.

Atopic dermatitis is divided into infantile, childhood and adult phases. In the infant and younger child, the lesions are more generalized than in the older child and adult. In the infantile phase, the condition is acute and subacute with erythema, edema, vesiculation, weeping and oozing. In the childhood and adult phases, it presents subacute and chronic features with erythema, papulation and lichenification, and a predilection for the flexural areas of the extremities. In addition, there is usually a generalized dryness of the skin, a characteristic facies manifested by periorbital discoloration and eyelid folds, white dermographism (upon stroking the skin a white line appears rather than the customary red line), and poor tolerance to various stresses such as cold, heat, humidity, trauma, infections and emotional tensions. Itching is a cardinal symptom.

It is not unusual to find the eruption localized to various parts of the body. Lesions confined to the lower legs and feet are more commonly seen in childhood and adolescence. The pattern of the disease in these areas presents special problems in diagnosis. One or more of the sites (e.g., the dorsa of the toes, the ankle or the soles) may be affected without other areas being involved. Thus, a chronic or recurrent dermatitis of the feet may be part of a more widespread dermatitis or a localized form of atopic dermatitis. It is necessary in these cases to question the patient regarding the familial background and past personal atopic history. It is also necessary to examine the patient for other atopic lesions or stigmata.

With children and adolescents, atopic dermatitis may manifest as lichenified patches around the ankles or behind the knees. With children particularly the dermatitis may become sharply localized to the dorsal aspect or to the tips of the toes (Fig. 5-21). The lesions may be confined to an area even as small as the dorsum of one toe. On the other hand, localized atopic dermatitis when complicated by injudi-

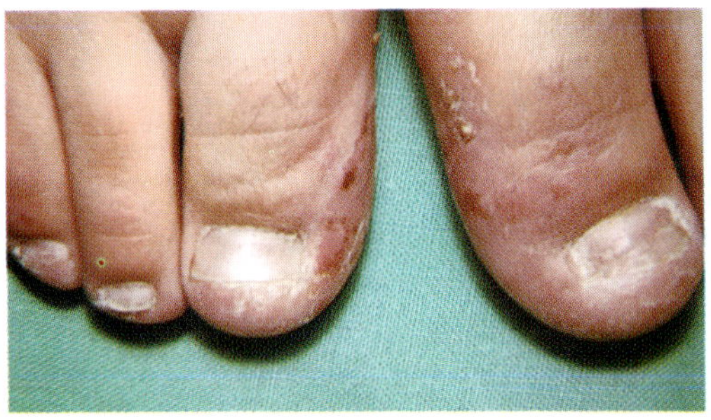

Fig. 5-21. Atopic dermatitis (juvenile type). The condition may often be misdiagnosed as a shoe box toe dermatitis.

cious treatment or over-treatment, infection or dyshidrosis can involve the soles, the legs and even become generalized. Toe involvement is usually the result of friction and irritation of ill-fitting shoes. The lesions and localization may resemble the picture of box toe dermatitis. However, reactions to patch tests with shoe materials are negative. While the soles are ordinarily not involved in atopic dermatitis, dyshidrosis frequently occurs here and causes difficulty in diagnosis (Fig. 5-22). Also, many cases which give the appearance of nummular eczema on the legs, in reality, are atopic dermatitis and must be treated as such.

Therapy of atopic dermatitis can be difficult even for the expert. It must be remembered that this is an inherited constitutional diathesis and therapy cannot change or cure this. Treatment should be directed to allay the itch-scratch symptoms and to control the process of eczematization and superimposed pyogenic infection (see treatment under contact dermatitis). Chronic lichenified patches respond well to coal tar pastes alone or over a previous application of corticosteroid creams. In children with toe involvement, avoidance of friction and irritation will remove a precipitating factor and along with the use of properly fitting shoes should afford considerable relief.

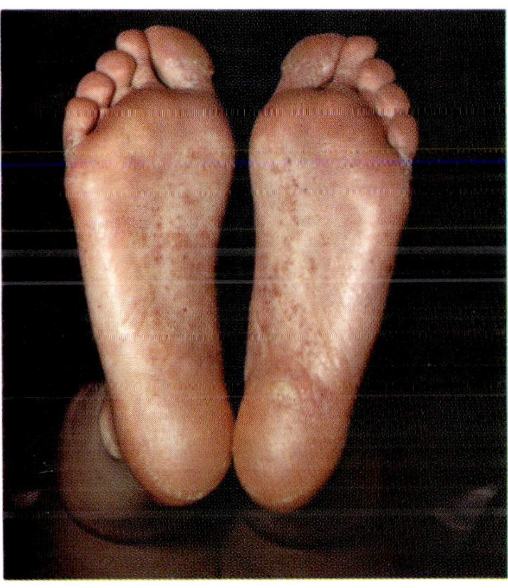

Fig. 5-22. Atopic dermatitis. The eruption was pronounced on the soles. At this site, differential diagnosis from hyperhidrosis is often difficult.

NUMMULAR ECZEMA

Nummular eczema presents a fairly typical clinical picture. Diagnosis depends on the characteristics of the lesions and distribution. Many hypotheses, as yet unsubstantiated, have been proposed regarding etiology. We consider the entity as a reaction pattern on a certain type of skin which is triggered by a variety of stimuli (viz., irritants, allergens, soap and water in association with microbial sensitization).

The lesions in nummular eczema, usually limited, are coin-shaped, varying in size from a dime to a palm-sized plaque. They are discrete with erythematous papulovesicular features, especially at the periphery. The centers often show a tendency for clearing. The vesicles are thin walled and tend to rupture easily, thus leading to oozing and crusting. The lesions may also present as isolated, mildly red plaques which are dry and scaly with superficial fissuring. Symmetrical distribution is characteristic: the dorsa of the hands and the extensor surfaces of forearms and legs. Less frequently, the shoulders, buttocks, face, breasts and nipples are involved. The disorder may begin as a single patch on a lower leg, usually on the calf or anterolateral aspect.

Nummular eczema is characterized by its persistence. After clearing, recurrences appear on exactly the same sites. The eruption tends to be worse in the cold weather. It is aggravated by soap and greasy applications and is associated with itching and burning.

The treatment of nummular eczema is trying both to the patient and physician. We have found the use of steroid creams alone or in association with a vioform-pine tar paste (3 percent vioform, 10 percent pine tar ointment in Lassar's paste), along with the administration of a broad spectrum antibiotic such as tetracycline (250 mg. q. i. d. for 3 to 5 days followed by 250 mg. every morning for several weeks) to be effective.

ASTEATOTIC ECZEMA

Under this heading we include eczematous pictures manifested by a dry, scaly or fissured state of the skin usually seen in elderly individuals. The skin usually presents a wrinkled or a "crazy-pavement" appearance (Fig. 5-23). Redness, edema, vesiculation and oozing may follow. Thickened and fissured lesions characterize the chronic stages of the disorder and itching is a very common complaint.

Various factors play a role in the etiology: an aging skin, the winter season, dryness of overheated homes, excessive cleansing with soaps, especially alkaline or bactericidal soaps, and friction from wearing apparel. The interplay between these factors results in an altered physiology of the skin. Soaps and cleansers may damage the epidermis and cause the production of an abnormal, horny layer which cannot serve as an efficient barrier and leads to dryness and chapping. If the process continues, the whole epidermis becomes involved with resultant eczematization. The lower extremities are common sites.

Treatment is simplified if the structural and functional integrity of the horny layer is restored and maintained. This is accomplished by lessening contact with irritants, the use of humidifiers, protection against exposure to cold, and the replacement of water in the skin by a hydration routine. A simple procedure is to have the patient soak the affected parts in lukewarm water for 10 to 15 minutes and, without drying the legs, apply an emollient such as white petrolatum or a vegetable fat such as Crisco or Spry and allow it to remain on the skin for 30 minutes, removing the excess with a towel. If inflammatory changes are present, corticosteroid creams or ointments are preferable. The routine can be repeated once or twice daily. The hydration helps to retain the normal suppleness of the skin.

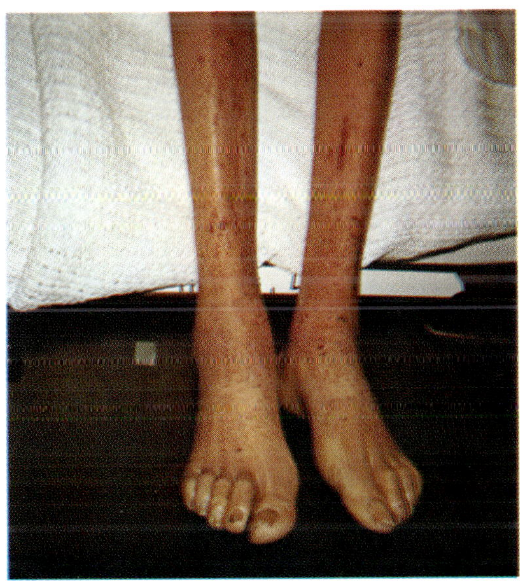

Fig. 5-23. Asteatotic eczema. The lower extremities are common sites for this problem.

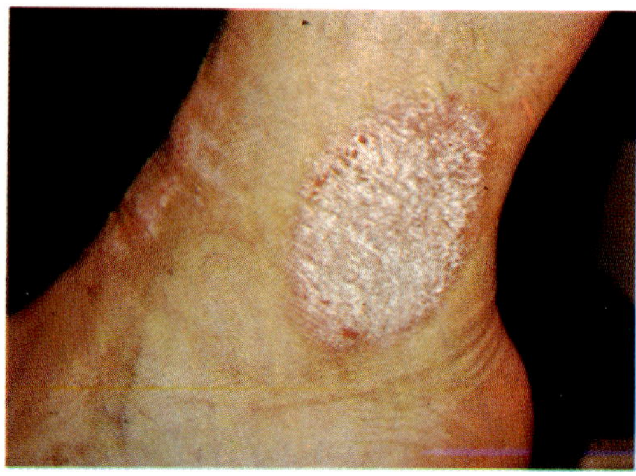

Fig. 5-24. Lichen simplex chronicus. The ankle is a common site for the itch-scratch picture.

LICHEN SIMPLEX CHRONICUS

Lichen simplex chronicus, also known as circumscribed neurodermatitis, occurs as variable sized patches in which lichenification is the distinctive feature (thickening and accentuation of the skin lines). The reaction arises on skin previously apparently normal and represents the response of the predisposed skin to repeated scratching and rubbing. External factors such as an insect bite or friction from wearing apparel may play a role in initiating the lesion. Emotions play a role in its perpetuation. The predominant symptom is intense pruritus which is often paroxysmal. Emotional events trigger the reaction. Scratching is the release mechanism. Thus the term "itch-scratch complex" is highly descriptive.

The fully developed lesion presents as a sharply demarcated patch of thickened skin, red and edematous during its early stage and subsequently dry, scaly, excoriated and hyperpigmented. A zone of grouped lichenoid papules surround the patch.

Lesions may occur in any area accessible to scratching. Favored sites on the lower extremity are the anterior surface of the leg especially just below the knee and on the ankles (Fig. 5-24). The typical lesion is a solitary patch. The condition may also occur on the soles. In this area it is often misdiagnosed as callus or psoriasis.

The objective in treatment is to break the itch-scratch cycle. The patient should be made to understand the causal relationships involved. Whatever therapy that can be directed to this end will help. We have found that discussing problems with the patient is far more useful than prescribing sedatives or tranquilizers.

Topical measures are very helpful with steroid cream as the treatment of choice. In the acute phase, simple compresses followed by the application of a steroid cream are most effective (see under contact dermatitis).

Occlusive dressings are preferable for chronic lesions, having a double purpose: They provide a barrier to prevent scratching and permit contact of the medication for longer periods of time. Modified Unna boots can be reapplied weekly. Tar pastes held in place with stockinette (an excellent simple form of dressing for the lower extremity) can be applied daily by the patient. Steroid creams applied under an occlusive plastic dressing can be changed once or twice daily.

Intralesional injections of corticosteroid suspensions (hydrocortisone or triamcinolone) are often used in lichen simplex. However, we do not recommend this modality for lesions on the ankle or foot because of a variety of adverse effects which we have observed. Severe lower back pain was experienced by several patients immediately following the injection. In others, ulcers (aseptic necrosis) developed at injection sites weeks after treatment.

If secondary infection is present, a topical antibiotic or an oral broad spectrum antibiotic may be required for a few days.

References

1. Rook, A. Wilkinson, D. S., and Ebling, F. J. G.: Textbook of Dermatology. Oxford, Blackwell Scientific Publications, 1968.

2. Montagna, W.: The Structure and Function of Skin. New York, Academic Press, 1962.

3. Samitz, M. H., and Gross, S.: Extraction by sweat of chromium from chrome-tanned leathers. J. Occup. Med., *2*:12, Jan., 1960.

4. Bloch, B.: The role of idiosyncrasy and allergy in dermatology. Arch. Derm. Syph., *19*:175, 1929.

5. Gaul, L. E., and Underwood, G. B.: Primary irritants and sensitizers used in fabrication of footwear. Arch. Derm. Syph., *60*:649, Nov., 1949.

6. Blank, I. H., and Miller, O. G.: A study of rubber adhesives in shoes as the cause of dermatitis of the feet. JAMA, *149*:1371, 1952.

7. Shatin, H., and Reisch, M.: Dermatitis of the feet due to shoes. Arch. Derm. Syph, *69*:651, June, 1954.

8. Morris, G. E.: "Chrome" dermatitis. Arch. Derm., *78*:612, Nov., 1958.

9. Fisher, A. A.: Some practical aspects of the diagnosis and management of shoe dermatitis. Arch. Derm., *79*:267, Mar., 1959.

10. Scutt, R. W. B.: Chrome sensitivity associated with tropical footwear in the Royal Navy. Brit. J. Derm., *78*:337, June, 1966.

11. Shatin, H., and Reisch, M.: Dermatitis of the feet due to shoes. Arch. Derm. Syph., *69*:651, June, 1954.

12. Calnan, C. D., and Sarkany, I.: Shoe dermatitis. Trans. St. John's Hosp. Derm. Soc., *43*:8-26, 1959.

13. Cronin, E.: Shoe dermatitis. Brit. J. Derm., *78*:617, Dec., 1966.

14. Gaul, L. E., and Underwood, G. B.: Primary irritants and sensitizers used in fabrication of footwear. Arch. Derm. Syph., *60*:649, Nov., 1949.

15. Shatin, H., and Reisch, M.: Dermatitis of the feet due to shoes. Arch. Derm. Syph., *69*:651, June, 1954.

16. *Ibid.*

17. Fisher, A. A.: Contact Dermatitis. Philadelphia, Lea & Febiger, 1967.

18. Brandao, F. N.: Shoe Dermatosis. Dermat. Ib. Lat. Am. (Eng. Ed.) Vol. II, 29, 1967.

19. Cronin, E.: Shoe dermatitis. Brit. J. Derm., *78*:617, Dec., 1966.

20. Fisher, A. A.: Some practical aspects of the diagnosis and management of shoe dermatitis. Arch. Derm., *79*:267, Mar., 1959.

21. Brandao, F. N.: Shoe Dermatosis. Dermat. Ib. Lat. Am. (Eng. Ed.), Vol. II, 29, 1967.

22. Malten, K. E., und van Aerssen, G. G. L.: Kontaktkzeme durch Leime bei Schuhmachern und Schujtragern. Berufsdermatosen, *10*:264, 1962.

23. deVries, H. R.: Allergic Dermatitis due to shoes. Dermatologica, Basel, *128*:68, 1964.

24. Suurmond, D., and Verspijck Mijnssen, G. A. W.: Allergic dermatitis due to shoes and a leather prothese. Dermatologica, *134*:371, 1967.

25. Cronin, E.: Shoe dermatitis. Brit. J. Derm., *78*:617, Dec., 1966.

26. Brandao, F. N.: Shoe Dermatosis. Dermat. Ib. Lat. Am. (Eng. Ed.), Vol. II, 29, 1967.

27. Samitz, M. H., and Gross, S.: Extraction by sweat of chromium from chrome-tanned leathers. J. Occup. Med., *2*:12, Jan., 1960.

28. Samitz, M. H., and Gross, S.: Effects of hexavalent and trivalent chromium compounds on the skin. Arch. Derm., *84*:404, Sept., 1961.

29. Scutt, R. W. B.: Chrome sensitivity associated with tropical footwear in the Royal Navy. Brit. J. Derm., *78*:337, June, 1966.

30. Fisher, A. A.: Contact Dermatitis. Philadelphia, Lea & Febiger, 1967.

31. Bett, D. C. G.: The potassium dichromate patch test. Trans. St. John's Hosp. Derm. Soc., *40*:40, 1958.

32. Samitz, M. H., and Gross, S.: Effects of hexavalent and trivalent chromium compounds on the skin. Arch. Derm., *84*:404, Sept., 1961.

33. Cronin, E.: Shoe dermatitis. Brit. J. Derm., *78*:617, Dec., 1966.

34. Calnan, C. D., and Sarkany, I.: Shoe dermatitis Trans. St. John's Hosp. Derm. Soc., *43*:8-26, 1959.

35. Fisher, A. A.: Contact Dermatitis. Philadelphia, Lea & Febiger, 1967.

36. Cronin, E.: Shoe dermatitis. Brit. J. Derm., *78*:617, Dec., 1966.

37. Fisher, A. A.: Contact Dermatitis. Philadelphia, Lea & Febiger, 1967.

38. Suurmond, D., and Verspijck Mijnssen, G. A. W.: Allergic dermatitis due to shoes and a leather prothese. Dermatologica, *134*:371, 1967.

39. Rook, A., Wilkinson, D. S., and Ebling, F. J. G.: Textbook of Dermatology. Philadelphia, F. A. Davis, 1968.

40. Suter, V. H.: Investigation of polyamide stocking eczema. Dermatologica, *130*:411, 1965.

41. Gibson, W. B.: Sweaty sock dermatitis. Clinical Pediat., *2*:175, 1963.

42. Rook, A., Wilkinson, D. S., and Ebling, F. J. G.: Textbook of Dermatology. Philadelphia, F. A. Davis, 1968.

43. Schamberg, I. L.: Allergic contact dermatitis to methyl and propyl paraben. Arch. Derm., *95*:626, June, 1967.

44. Provost, T. T., and Jillson, O. F.: Ethylenediamine contact dermatitis. Arch. Derm., *96*:231, Sept., 1967.

45. Spencer, M. C.: Herbicide dermatitis. JAMA, *198*:1307, Dec., 1966.

46. Ross. J. B.: Rubber boot dermatitis in Newfoundland: A survey of 30 patients. Canad. Med. Ass. J., *100*:13, 1969.

47. Fisher, A. A.: Contact Dermatitis. Philadelphia, Lea & Febiger, 1967.

48. Hack, M.: Chemical and mechanical etiology of shoe dermatitis. Cutis, *6*:529, May, 1970.

6

Papulosquamous Diseases

PSORIASIS

Psoriasis is a common disorder which is known to be inherited as an autosomal dominant with irregular penetrance. It is characterized by its epidermal kinetics and by certain histologic features. Its clinical morphology is distinctive.

The etiology of psoriasis is unknown. Endocrine, infectious, metabolic, and neurogenic factors have been considered. However, there are no conclusive scientific data to confirm these theories.

Kinetics. The epidermal turnover time, (i.e., the time required for a basal cell to reach the surface and be cast off) is reduced from the normal 28 to 30 days to 3 to 4 days. This implies an intense metabolic activity which has been demonstrated by various technics.

Histology. Psoriasis includes both epidermal and dermal alterations: (1) an increased and abnormal horny layer (parakeratosis); (2) the migration of polymorphonuclear leukocytes into the horny layer which produces characteristic microabscesses (Munro's abscesses); and (3) dilatation of dermal papillary capillaries with a surrounding round cell infiltration. The clinical appearance of the psoriatic lesion is determined by the predominance of one or another of these changes.

Clinical Findings. The abnormal horny layer gives rise to the distinctive scale characteristic of the psoriatic lesion. The silvery appearance of the scale is due to air pockets in the horny layer. The microabscesses in the horny layer are not apparent on gross examination. Dilatation of the capillaries in the tips of the elongated dermal papillae give the vivid red color to the psoriatic lesion.

Two clinical hallmarks of the disease are the (1) Auspitz sign in which manual removal of scale exposes the capillaries through the thinned suprapapillary portion of the stratum malpighii and results in minute bleeding points, and the (2) Koebner phenomenon which refers to extension or aggravation of the psoriatic lesion after local trauma such as scarification or scratching. The Koebner phenomenon is not diagnostic but only suggestive evidence of psoriasis.

The forms of psoriasis are many. Those most commonly seen on the lower extremities are: (1) regular psoriasis on the legs, (2) psoriatic keratoderma on the soles, (3) interdigital psoriasis, (4) pustular psoriasis, localized to the palms and the soles, (5) psoriasis of the nails, and (6) psoriatic arthropathy.

Psoriasis en Plaque. It is rarely seen only on the lower extremities but is usually part of a more extensive process involving upper extremities,

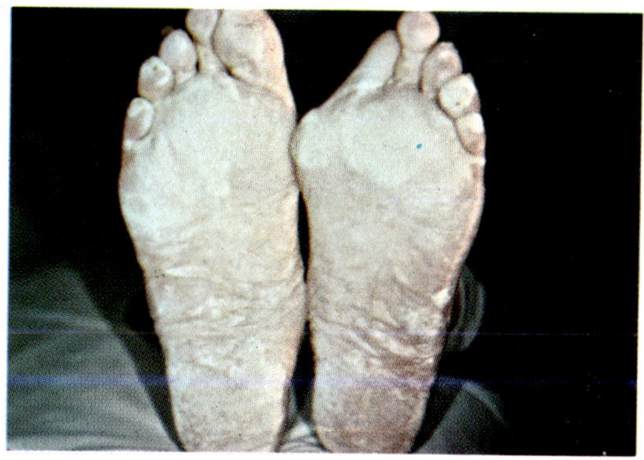

Fig. 6-1. Psoriasis on the plantar surfaces.

trunk and scalp. It is manifested by well-demarcated erythematous plaques capped by white scales. Involvement tends to be symmetrical. It is particularly chronic and difficult to manage. Lesions on the lower extremities respond to therapy last and least.

Psoriatic Keratoderma. It presents as marginated hyperkeratotic plaques and is an especially protracted and rebellious form of psoriasis. This form may involve the palms as well as the soles. Palmoplantar psoriasis displays various degrees of erythema, hyperkeratosis and fissures. It is almost always bilateral and symmetrical extending in well-defined erythematosquamous plaques and exfoliating in dry, friable lamellae. Massive yellowish or greyish keratoderma due to a greatly thickened horny layer is often seen with deep painful fissures (Fig. 6-1).

Interdigital Psoriasis. This entity otherwise known as "white psoriasis" was described by Waisman.[1] Five percent of psoriasis patients are supposedly affected. The lesions are marked by whitish hyperkeratosis accompanied by maceration and fissuring located between the toes or at their bases (Figs. 6-2, 6-3). It is usually accompanied by other localizations, but as an isolated finding it must be differentiated from interdigital dermatophytosis and erythrasma. The histology is diagnostic of psoriasis.

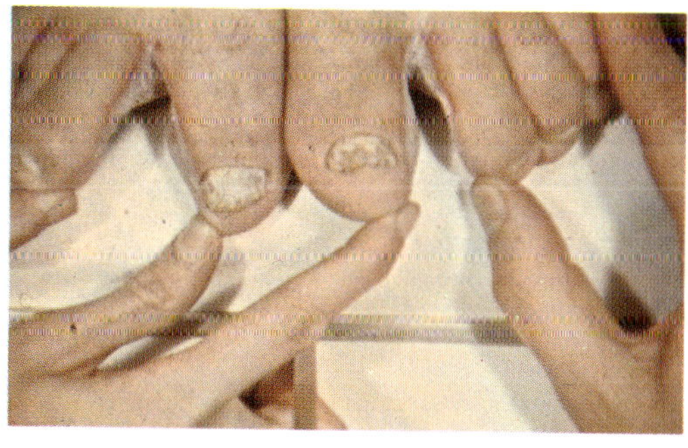

Fig. 6-2. "White psoriasis" of webs of toes. Patient also had psoriasis of toenails.

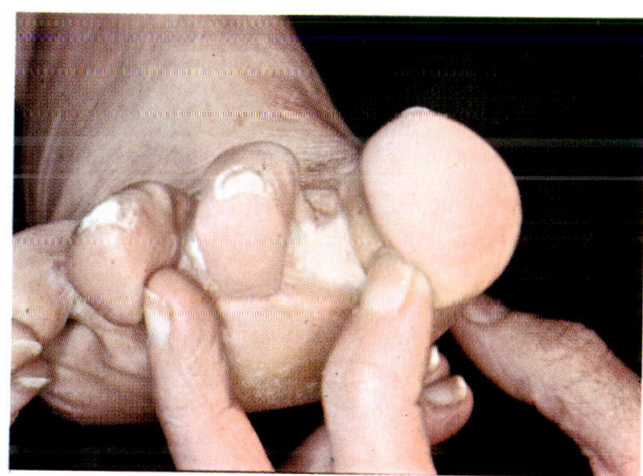

Fig. 6-3. "White psorasis" close-up.

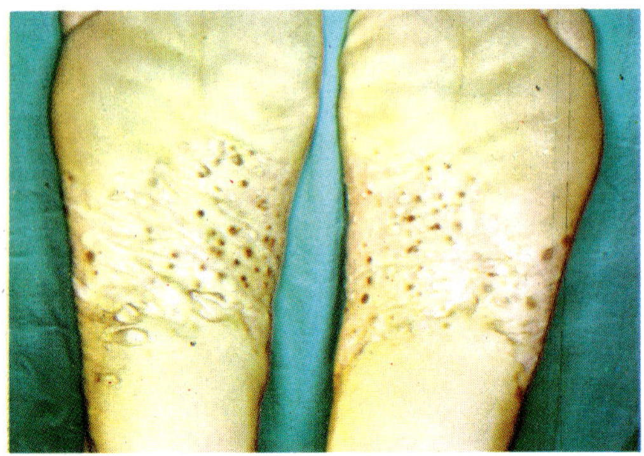

Fig. 6-4. Typical lesions of pustular psoriasis of soles.

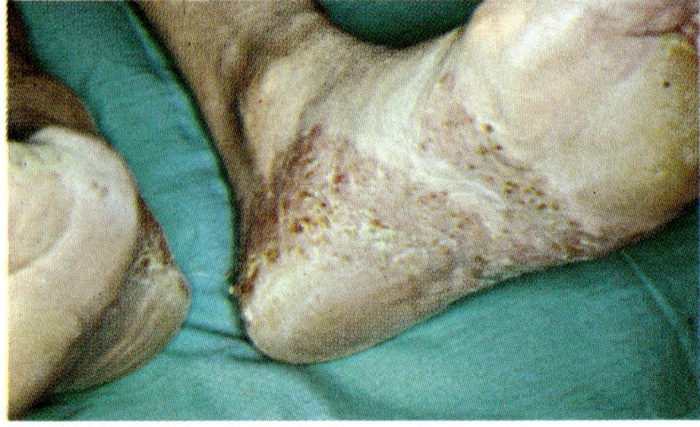

Fig. 6-5. Pustular psoriasis of soles.

Pustular Psoriasis. It is a morphologic variation of psoriasis. A localized form involves the palms and soles. This type often occurs in the absence of typical psoriasis elsewhere, but may occur concomitantly. The eruption, almost always bilateral and symmetrical, usually starts on the internal aspect of the plantar arch (Figs. 6-4, 6-5). Occasionally, the initial attack may be characterized by showers of pustules which are sterile. They involute slowly to form hard, brownish squamous crusts. Recurrences of pustules may be preceded by a smarting sensation. Recurrences produce scaly and parakeratotic surfaces before exfoliating. Histopathology shows changes of psoriasis.

Psoriasis of the Nails. Psoriatic nail changes occur with or without skin involvement, in 10 to 60 percent of psoriatics. The nail changes are analogous to those of psoriasis of the skin. Biochemical changes are similar to those in psoriatic scales. Nail abnormalities range from simple stippling or punctate pitting and from a yellow, opaque discoloration with disfigurement and terminal crumbling with hyperkeratotic debris to shortening, partial destruction and detachment of the nails. Periungual changes, diffuse redness, swelling and desquamation, are frequent.

Differential diagnosis of psoriasis of the nails should include onychomycosis, eczematous dermatitides, lichen planus, occupational or traumatic changes, alopecia areata and various onychodystrophies.

Psoriatic Arthropathy. The psoriatic type of arthritis is usually seen in diffuse forms of psoriasis. The psoriasis and arthritis usually wax and wane together. Distal interphalangeal joints of the hands and feet are most commonly involved. The affliction is asymmetrical, and the deformities are unlike the classical changes in rheumatoid arthritis. Absence of rheumatoid factor differentiates the latter.

Treatment

Our present limited understanding of the pathogenesis of psoriasis precludes a cure. Meanwhile, a rational therapeutic approach should utilize measures to correct the known tissue abnormalities. In our experience, there is little need of systemic medication for ordinary psoriasis. Control of the psoriatic eruption is obtained by suitable topical regimens which include such measures as hydration baths, tar and ultraviolet light combinations (Goeckerman regimen), and externally applied medications fitted to the requirement of the individual patient.

Local therapy is still the safest method of treatment. Acute types of psoriasis do best with corticosteroids (Valisone 0.1 percent, Kenalog 0.025 percent, Synalar 0.025 percent, Cordran 0.025 percent) under occlusion or when applied on wet skin. Occlusion enhances penetration. Chronic types can be benefited with inunctions of tar-ammoniated mercury-salicylic acid ointments. The use of ultraviolet light with topical tar (Goeckerman regimen) has the distinct advantage of producing longer remission than most other modalities. In patients resistant to previous therapy, we prefer the Ingram method which uses Lassar's paste with 0.1 percent anthralin and 0.4 percent salicylic acid applied after a coal-tar bath, then talc and stockinette.

Castellani's paint may be used in fissured lesions and interdigital psoriasis.

Intralesional steroids (preferably triamcinolone in a concentration of 5.0 mg. per cubic centimeter) are effective for localized lesions; however, we do not recommend its use for lesions on the ankle or foot because of adverse reactions which we have observed when used on these sites (see under lichen simplex chronicus).

Ionizing radiation inhibits cellular proliferation and can be useful in controlling the psoriatic lesion. However, the potential dangers of these ionizing rays has been well established and x-rays should be used with caution in this chronic disease. We are against its use.

Systemic therapy offers no conclusive scientific data to confirm the efficacy of hormone therapy, fat free, low cholesterol, low protein, low tryptophan, or low amino acid taurine diets, dietary supplements such as vitamins, wheat germ, pancreatic enzymes or anti-infective agents.

Many dermatologists do not favor systemic steroids for psoriasis under any circumstances. The risk of complications such as exfoliation and likelihood of serious exacerbation on withdrawal of medication are too great to take. Others limit their use to severe cases of psoriatic arthritis or psoriatic erythroderma.

Methotrexate given orally or parenterally has proved effective in many cases of psoriasis resistant to other modalities of treatment. However, it is a potent antimetabolite of folic acid and its use must be weighed carefully because of its toxic effects on multiple organ systems. The only existing indication for its use in psoriasis is the presence of grave emotional disability ensuing from this disease or severe disabling psoriatic arthritis.

References

1. Waisman, M.: Interdigital psoriasis ("white psoriasis"). Arch. Derm., *84*: 733, 1961.

LICHEN PLANUS

Lichen planus is an inflammatory dermatosis of unknown origin, starting insidiously or suddenly. Psychogenic factors may be involved and it may mimic a drug eruption (atabrine). It runs a sluggish course and often is recurrent. Although the eruption may be asymptomatic, more often there is pruritus of variable degree.

Characteristic lesions occur in variable patterns both on the skin and mucous membranes. The diagnostic lesion is a small, flat-topped, polygonal, violaceous papule that later becomes brownish and may leave deep pigmentation. Other lesions of lichen planus may be annular or centrally umbilicated. The surface may show a whitish network called Wickham's striae. Papules may be arranged in patches, in linear or annular configuration or confluent in large plaques. Common sites of involvement are the flexor aspects of the arms and extensor surface of the lower extremity, the buccal mucosa and the penis.

Most cases of lichen planus last 6 to 9 months; there are few forms of therapy that alter its natural course. The prospect of permanent remission in lichen planus is much better than in psoriasis.

Histologically, the features of lichen planus are diagnostic regardless of the site of involvement or the clinical type. There is hyperkeratosis, a thickened stratum granulosum, irregular acanthosis and liquefaction necrosis of the basal layer. A band of cellular infiltrate (mainly lymphocytes with a few histiocytes) presses against the epidermis, hugging and invading it.

VARIATIONS OF LICHEN PLANUS ON THE LOWER EXTREMITY

The most persistent form of lichen planus is hypertrophic lichen planus that classically involves the shins and ankles. Such lesions persist for many more months and even years than in ordinary lichen planus. The lesions are thickened, warty, hypertrophic plaques covered with fine adherent scales. The patches vary in size and configuration, are reddish brown or purplish, and are characterized by their chronicity (Fig. 6-6). The lesions usually itch severely; burning and stinging are less common complaints. Careful inspection of the lesions will usually reveal a typical papule. When hypertrophic lichen planus lesions eventually involute, corresponding areas of depigmentation and some degree of atrophy may remain. The differentiation from lichen amyloidosus and from lichen simplex chronicus may be difficult.

Lesions of lichen planus of the soles are usually situated along the sides rather than the center of the sole. Their color may range from pink to yellow. Here they present as papules or nodules (Fig. 6-7), less often because of coalescence and thickening, they resemble calluses.

Nail changes[1,2] vary from longitudinal striations, ridging, splitting and midline fissures to progressive atrophy with eventual total destruction. Most characteristic is the paper-like thinning of the nail plate in association with an overgrowth of the cuticle and its subsequent attachment to the nail plate (pterygium formation), the great toenails being

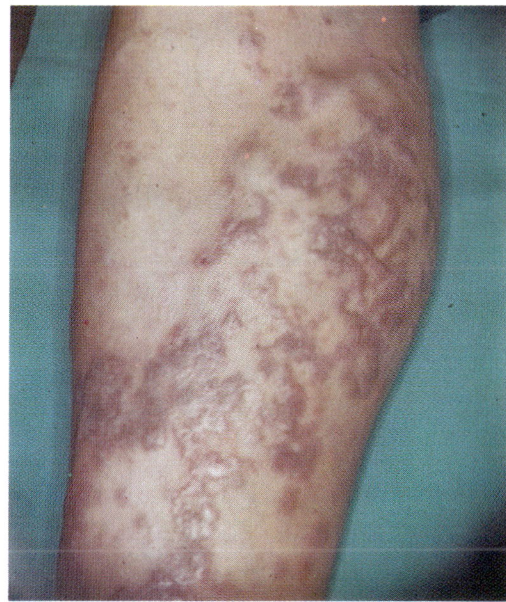

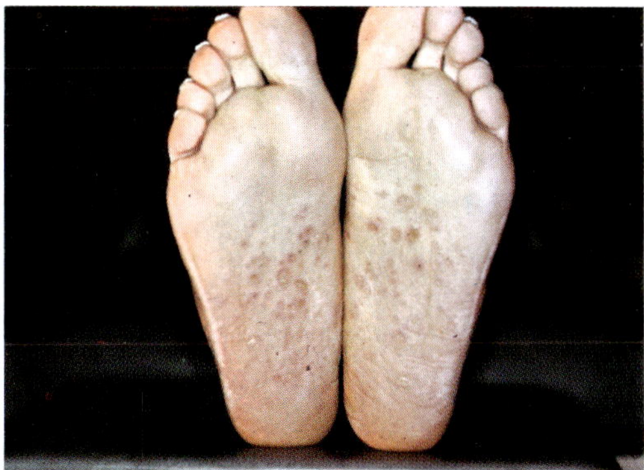

Fig. 6-7. Lichen planus of the soles.

Fig. 6-6. Lichen planus. The lesions show features of early hypertrophic lichen planus.

most often affected in this way. The minor nail changes are temporary but the more severe forms are often permanent. Lichen planus of the nails must be differentiated from onychomycosis, psoriasis, and from nail changes due to impaired peripheral circulation or following trauma.

Permanent loss of nails due to lichen planus has been reported by Cornelius III and Shelley.[3] In this unusual case, a 60-year-old woman showed permanent loss of her toenails with scaling and superficial erosion of the nail bed and matrix. The unusual feature here was that the surrounding skin was normal except for an erythematous scaly dermatitis on the big toe. The patient gave a history of recurrent, painful, superficial ulcerations occurring in the areas of the toenail, which healed without complications. The fingernails were normal. Hyperkeratotic scaling of the edges of the soles and a few follicular keratotic papules on the dorsa of the feet were the only other skin findings. Biopsy of the nail matrix of an involved toe showed the typical histology of lichen planus. The dermatitis responded to topical steroids and Castellani's paint.

An unusual syndrome of lichen planus has been reported, characterized by bullae and ulcerations confined to the feet and toes, permanent loss of toenails, and a cicatricial alopecia of the scalp.[4,5,6] Distinctive are the chronic, painful and disabling ulcerations of the feet which present a problem of diagnosis. The toes showed bleeding and the granulating ulcers were surrounded by atrophic depigmented skin.

Treatment

Because the etiology of lichen planus is still unknown, treatment is mainly symptomatic and often unsatisfactory.

Antipruritic lotions and corticosteroid creams help relieve itching. We prefer applying the latter on the wet skin. Fluorinated steroid creams under occlusive plastic films can be beneficial. Occasionally intralesional injections of triamcinolone are useful and tar or icthammol pastes can be used.

At times, the patient requires rest and relief of tensions, thus, mild sedatives or antihistaminics are helpful. There is no indication for systemic corticosteroids in the localized forms of lichen planus on the lower extremities and there is no rationale in old remedies such as bismuth or arsenic.

References

1. Ronchese, F.: Nail in lichen planus. Arch. Derm., *91*:347, Apr., 1965.

2. Samman, P. D.: The nails in lichen planus. Brit. J. Derm., *73*:288, July, 1961.

3. Cornelius III, C. E., and Shelley, W. B.: Permanent anonychia due to lichen planus. Arch. Derm., *96*:434, 1967.

4. Corsi, H.: Lichen planus associated with atrophy of nail matrix and hair follicles on scalp. Proc. Roy. Soc. Med., *30*:198, 1936-37.

5. Pierini, L. E., Abulafia, J., and Barnatan, M.: El liquen como factor de exoniquia definitiva. Arch Argent. Derm., *4*:287, Sept., 1954.

6. Cram, D. L., Kierland, R., R., and Winkelmann, R. K.: Ulcerative lichen planus of the feet: bullous variant with hair and nail lesions. Arch. Derm., *93*:692, June, 1966.

PITYRIASIS RUBRA PILARIS

Pityriasis rubra pilaris is a rare, chronic, mildly pruritic, inflammatory disease, characterized by fine, acuminate, horny, follicular papules. The etiology is unknown but some feel that it is an inherited, simple autosomal, heterozygous condition. The papules may be preceded by or superimposed upon a seborrhea of the scalp and face. There is often a striking keratoderma of the palms and soles. This unusually thick keratinous, salmon-yellow scaling of the palms and soles is called the "keratodermic sandal of pityriasis rubra pilaris." There is a slow evolution of widespread areas of follicular papules involving not only extremities, but also the trunk and face. Differential diagnosis must include phrynoderma (vitamin A deficiency), psoriasis and exfoliative erythroderma. Diagnostic are the black, horny, follicular plugs in hair follicles one sees on the dorsa of the fingers. "White islands" of uninvolved skin may be seen within red papulosquamous plaques.[1] Erythematous scaling plaques may resemble psoriasis and in some cases there may be exfoliation. The keratodermic sandal of pityriasis rubra pilaris is often difficult to differentiate from the heritable plantar keratodermas.

Histologically, pityriasis rubra pilaris shows follicular and diffuse hyperkeratosis with spotty parakeratosis. The epidermis shows mild irregular acanthosis and there is liquefactive degeneration of the basal cell layer. A mild chronic perivascular inflammatory infiltrate is found in the dermis.

Treatment

Approximately 50 percent of patients become symptom free after an average duration of 2 to 3 years of the disease regardless of the therapy used.[2] It is therefore difficult to evaluate the effectiveness of therapy or, in fact, whether treatment is useful.

Vitamin A, 150,000 units daily orally or by intramuscular injections proved to be favorable in some cases. Prolonged and massive doses (Aquasol A, 500,000 units daily) together with moderate doses of hydroxychloroquine (Plaquenil 400 mg. daily) have been reported as improving the keratoderma of palms and soles, with no improvement of the rest of the body.[3]

A case report by Waldorf and Hambrick, Jr.[4] described a patient with pityriasis rubra pilaris, myasthenia gravis and hypovitaminosis A. Among other findings, the patient had progressive yellow thickening of her palms and soles which diminished considerably after 10 weeks' therapy with water-miscible vitamin A, 200,000 units orally b. i. d. Topical 2 percent vitamin A methyl ester in an emollient base tried previously was unsuccessful. The serum vitamin A level rose to normal after one week of therapy.

Methotrexate, preferably by daily small doses, has brought about a marked clinical improvement which was maintained when treatment was stopped.[5] The folic acid antagonist carries with it the potential of

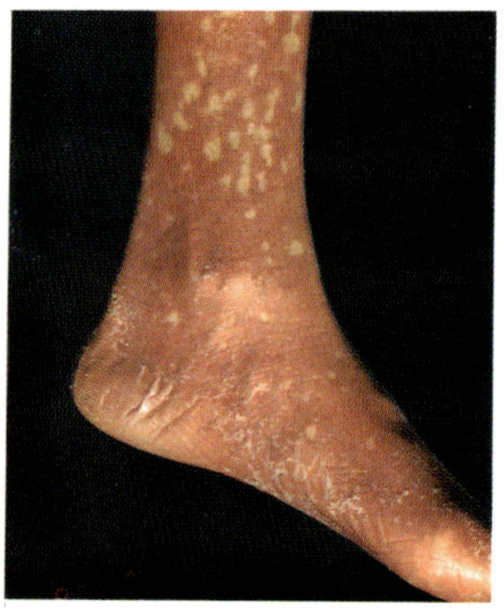

Fig. 6-8. Pityriasis rubra pilaris. The keratodermic sandal has involuted considerably with vitamin A under occlusion. Note the "white islands" of uninvolved skin within red papulosquamous plaques.

severe side-effects. Its use should be restricted to severe expressions of the disease which cannot be controlled by conventional therapy.

The keratoderma of the soles may require only keratolytic ointments and lubricating agents; much more effective has been the topical use of vitamin A acid[6,7] and vitamin A alcohol.[8] We have seen a dramatic response with vitamin A acid (0.1 to 0.5 percent) under occlusion (Fig. 6-8).

References

1. Sidi, E., Zagula-Mally, Z. W., and Hincky, M.: Psoriasis. Springfield, (Ill.), Charles C Thomas, 1968.

2. Davidson, C. L., Jr., Winkelmann, R. K., and Kierland, R. R.: Pityriasis rubra pilaris. Arch. Derm., *100*:175, Aug., 1969.

3. Watt, T. L., and Jillson, O. F.: Pityriasis rubra pilaris: penicillin and antituberculous drugs as possible therapeutic agents. Arch. Derm., *92*:428, 1965.

4. Waldorf, D. S., and Hambrick, G. W., Jr.: Vitamin A-responsive pityriasis rubra pilaris with myasthenia gravis. Arch. Derm., *92*:424, 1965.

5. Chernosky, M. E.: Pityriasis Rubra Pilaris: Treatment with methotrexate. Paper read at 28th Annual Meeting of Amer. Acad. of Derm., Bal Harbour, Florida, Dec. 11, 1969.

6. Beer, P.: Studies on the effect of vitamin A acid. Dermatologica, *124*:192, 1962.

7. Stuttgen, G.: Local treatment of keratoses with vitamin A acid. Dermatologica, *124*:65, 1962.

8. Lamar, L. M., and Gaethe, G.: Pityriasis rubra pilaris. Arch. Derm., *89*:515, 1964.

7

Nodose Lesions

NODOSE LESIONS

While it is always useful to arrange a group of diseases in a logical manner to facilitate understanding, we believe that such systemization is not possible with the nodose lesions of the leg. Therefore, we will simply list the clinical syndromes and discuss each one in turn.

NODOSE LESIONS OF THE LEGS

1. Erythema nodosum
2. Erythema induratum
3. Nodular vasculitis
4. Subacute nodular migratory panniculitis
5. Weber-Christian disease
6. Lipogranulomatosis of Rothmann-Makai
7. Subcutaneous nodular fat necrosis in association with pancreatic diseases

ERYTHEMA NODOSUM

Erythema nodosum is a reaction pattern of the skin which can be elicited by a wide variety of stimuli and embraces several etiologies. The lesions consist of red, tender, painful nodules, usually on the pretibial portions of the lower legs (Fig. 7-1), infrequently developing on the arms or elsewhere. The nodules tend to appear in crops, with each

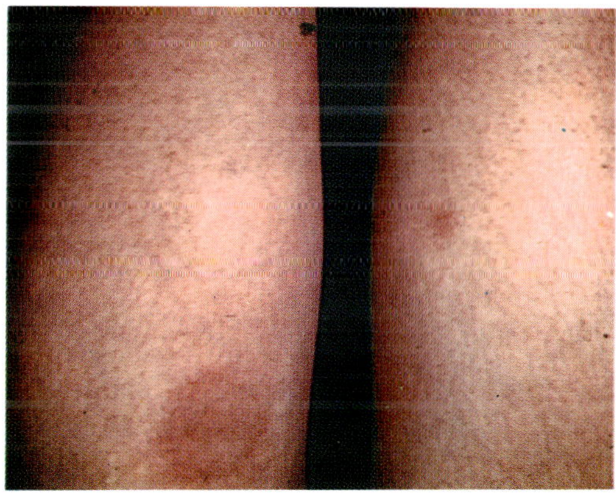

Fig. 7-1. Erythema nodosum.

episode associated with mild systemic symptoms of fever, malaise, and joint or muscle pain. They never ulcerate and characteristically undergo spontaneous slow involution over a period of several weeks.

The idiopathic form of erythema nodosum usually has an abrupt onset accompanied by fever and arthralgias. The nodose lesions are relatively few in number, are almost all of the same age, and evolve through a series of color changes closely mimicking an absorbing hematoma.[1]

Symptomatic or secondary erythema nodosum displays lesions which are not as uniform in appearance as in idiopathic erythema nodosum, and their course is more variable. Recurrences are common if the provoking drug is administered or the disease state recurs.[2]

Because of their high incidence, streptococcic infections are probably the most common cause of erythema nodosum. Other diseases which may underlie the eruption are tuberculosis, sarcoidosis, deep fungal infections (histoplasmosis, coccidioidomycosis), ulcerative colitis, rheumatic fever, lymphogranuloma venereum, syphilis, scarlet fever, chancroid, meningococcemia, cat scratch disease, leprosy, and lymphoblastomas. It is not unusual for the lesions of erythema nodosum to be the only manifestation of an occult systemic disease. Proper recognition of the possible significance of the eruption can lead to comprehensive study of the patient and an etiologic diagnosis.[3]

Erythema nodosum may also be a manifestation of drug sensitivity, especially to iodides, salicylates, sulfonamides, barbiturates, penicillin, and bromides. Recently, reports have appeared of patients who developed erythema nodosum from oral contraceptive pills.[4,5] It has been postulated that the progestational agent may be the causative factor.[6]

On histologic examination, a scattered infiltrate extending along septa between fat cells in the upper subcutaneous tissue is seen. Abscess formation or necrosis do not occur. Blood vessels, particularly the larger veins, may show invasion of the walls by an inflammatory infiltrate and marked endothelial proliferation.[7] The histologic features of erythema nodosum, though distinctive, are not those of the underlying disease.

Therapy should not be directed toward the erythema nodosum itself. If a drug sensitivity is suspected, the possible culprit should be withdrawn. If study reveals one of the underlying diseases known to incite erythema nodosum, the basic disease should be treated appropriately. Idiopathic erythema nodosum is a self-limiting disease which resolves spontaneously.

ERYTHEMA INDURATUM

Lengthy debate has revolved about the use of the term erythema induratum. The dilemma centers about those cases of erythema induratum which are classical clinically and histologically, but where no acid-fast bacilli can be found in the biopsy specimens, or can active internal tuberculosis be demonstrated. Some authors believe that the

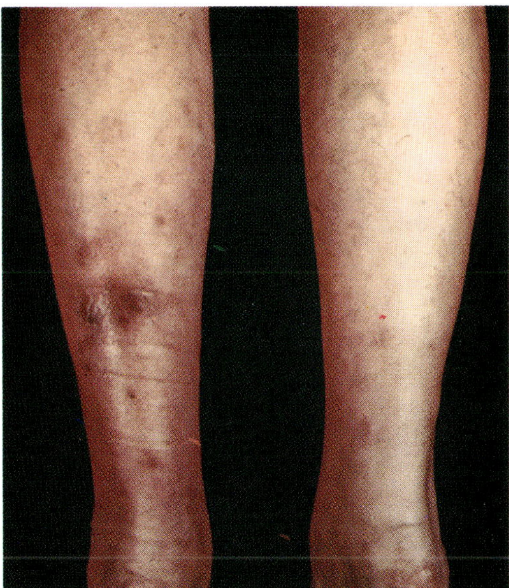

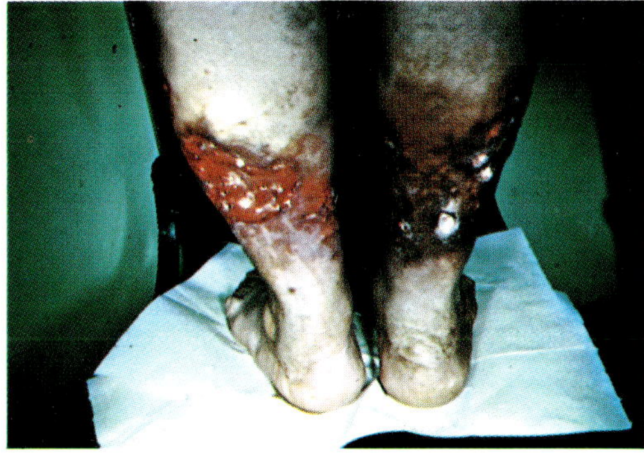

Fig. 7-3. Erythema induratum with severe ulcerations.

Fig. 7-2. Erythema induratum.

term erythema induratum denotes a tuberculous id and an internal mycobacterial infection must be assumed even if it cannot be found.[8] But Irgang pointed out[9] a histologically proved tuberculid requires adequate antituberculous therapy to eradicate the internal infection even if it cannot be located.

Other investigators think that erythema induratum is a descriptive term only and does not imply a specific etiology.[10] There is no question that nontuberculous disorders may precisely simulate erythema induratum clinically. The differential diagnosis includes erythema nodosum, nodular allergic vasculitis, gummatous syphilid, nodose lesions secondary to iodides and bromides, panniculitis, and thrombophlebitis.

Thus, erythema induratum "may well be a syndrome having a number of causes as yet undetermined."[11]

Classical erythema induratum, also known as Bazin's disease and tuberculosis cutis indurativa, is a notoriously chronic, recurrent syndrome predominant among young, adult women. The lesions begin as deep subcutaneous nodules on indistinct infiltrated areas and gradually come nearer to the surface, forming bluish-red nodules or plaques (Fig. 7-2). Necrosis develops, often leading to the formation of ulcers (Fig. 7-3); however, the nodose lesions may resorb without the appearance of ulcers. In either case, atrophic scarring is the ultimate result.

The lesions are usually bilateral and tend to be symmetrical. The nodules evolve through various stages. The nodules, plaques, and ulcers most often occur on the calves of the legs, but rarely appear on the thighs and arms. Though most authors report that sensory symptoms are usually insignificant, Feiwel and Munro[12] described significant pain associated with the nodose lesions and increased discomfort when ulcers appeared.

Histopathologically, erythema induratum shows tuberculoid structures, caseation necrosis, and extensive infiltration and thickening of the larger arteries and veins. The changes are limited to the lower dermis and subcutis in the earlier lesions, but necrosis in older lesions may extend to the epidermis and lead to ulceration. Compared to erythema nodosum, erythema induratum has caseation necrosis, extensive tuberculoid and abscess formation, none of which occurs in erythema nodosum. The infiltrate of Bazin's disease is also more extensive and massive.[13]

It is generally agreed that the preferred antituberculous chemotherapeutic agent is INH, administered in daily doses of 300 mg. for 9 to 12 months. Occasionally PAS is also given, but only as an adjunct to INH. A dose of PAS 12.5 gm. combined with INH 200 to 260 mg. daily for 9 months or more has been reported as yielding excellent results.[14]

Interestingly, Feiwel and Munro also noted that many patients who did not have systemic symptoms of tuberculosis improved and gained weight on antituberculous therapy.

NODULAR VASCULITIS

In a series of articles during the first decade of this century, Whitfield dissociated a group of nontuberculous conditions from erythema induratum. One of these conditions, initially described by Whitfield under the name of nontuberculous erythema induratum, is now recognized as nodular vasculitis. This term was introduced in 1945 by Montgomery, O'Leary, and Barker[15] to describe a chronic, painful, usually nonulcerative, nodular eruption on the legs of middle-aged or older women. The lesions often coalesced to form plaques and, on occasion, a plaque was the initial lesion. The nodules often simulate erythema nodosum or erythema induratum, but usually are sufficiently distinct for clinical differentiation (Fig. 7-4).

Histologically, nodular vasculitis resembles the late stage of erythema nodosum, but exhibits a greater degree of vascular involvement, including vessels of a large diameter.

The etiology of nodular vasculitis remains unknown at the present time. However, several factors suggest that an immune mechanism may

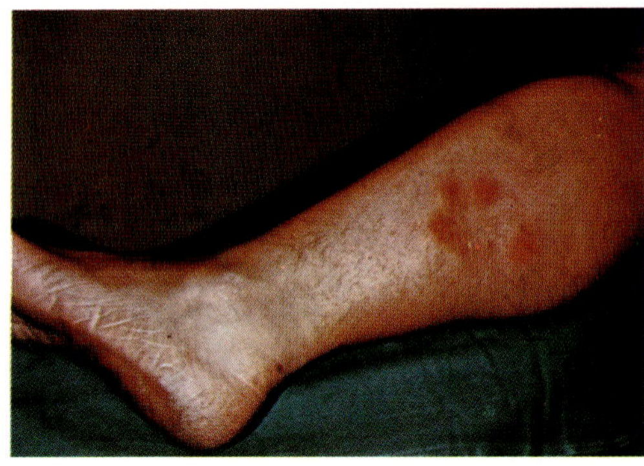

Fig. 7-4. Nodular vasculitis.

be operative, and a recent study[16] has lent further support to this possibility by demonstrating immune globulins at the sites of fibrinoid necrosis of vessels.

SUBACUTE NODULAR MIGRATORY PANNICULITIS

In 1956 Vilanova and Aguade described subacute nodular migratory panniculitis. More recently, Perry and Winkelmann[17] reviewed 14 cases diagnosed histologically as migratory panniculitis. The syndrome occurs most commonly in middle-aged women who develop discrete nontender nodules, usually on the anterolateral aspect of the leg. The lesions usually affect only one leg initially and enlarge rapidly in 1 to 3 weeks to attain a diameter of 10 to 20 cm.

The outer, extending margin of the lesion is bright red while the resolving portion has a yellowish tint. The plaques usually become quite indurated, at times almost scleroderma-like, with a mottled consistency, and persist for months or several years (Fig. 7-5). The erythrocyte sedimentation rate is elevated in most cases. Ulceration of the lesions is rare.

The histologic picture is characteristic, but not specific. The pathologic changes are limited to the septa between fat lobules but there is no involvement of the fat lobules themselves or of the blood vessels. In the septa are numerous histiocytes with giant cells and a mild lymphocytic inflammatory reaction. Occasionally hemorrhage also is present. Though Vilanova and Aguade described a capillaritis, Perry and Winkelmann believe that the picture seen is more compatible with a proliferative reaction of vessels than with an inflammatory reaction.

The lesions of subacute nodular migratory panniculitis respond quite readily to systemic iodide administration for reasons which are not clear. The etiology of this interesting condition is unknown.

Perry and Winkelmann point out that on clinical examination the plaque of subacute nodular migratory panniculitis may mimic any of the other chronic inflammatory lesions of the legs. However, the characteristic history of "an asymptomatic unilateral indurated red plaque of the leg that has developed in a woman by peripheral growth in all directions from a single initial nodule, but at the same time shows central resolution" should suggest the diagnosis.[18]

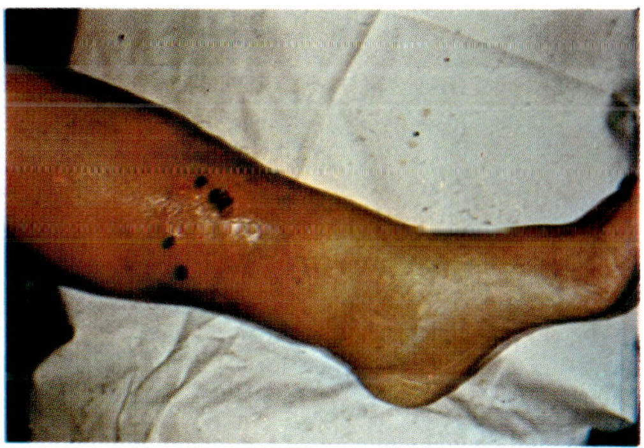

Fig. 7-5. Subacute nodular migratory panniculitis.

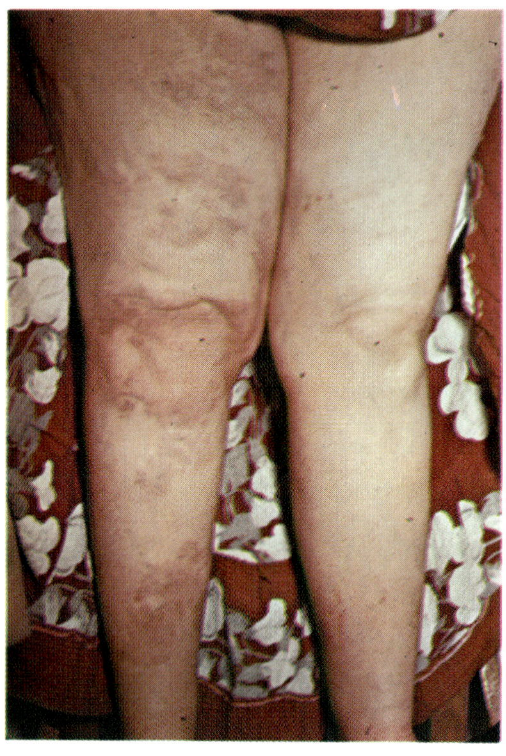

Fig. 7-6. Weber-Christian disease.

WEBER-CHRISTIAN DISEASE

Also known as relapsing febrile nodular nonsuppurative panniculitis, or simply as nodular panniculitis, this disease state consists of crops of tender, painful subcutaneous nodules, usually on the thigh or buttocks but may occur at any subcutaneous location. The nodules are of variable size and present as inflammatory lesions with overlying erythematous skin (Fig. 7-6). The disease occurs much more often in women than men and is particularly frequent in obese women between 20 and 40 years of age.

During an acute attack, the patient often has fever, and each attack of nodular panniculitis may last for a month or more. By and large the nodules do not break down or ulcerate. The fat necrosis which occurs during the acute episodes leaves the affected skin sites depressed and pigmented after the inflammatory changes regress.

The etiology of this condition is unknown. Histologically Weber-Christian nodular panniculitis shows a nonspecific fat necrosis with numerous lymphocytes throughout the fat. Secondary vascular inflammatory involvement is common.

The clinical differential diagnosis includes erythema nodosum, erythema induratum, thrombophlebitis, nodular vasculitis, nonspecific traumatic fat necrosis, subcutaneous rheumatic nodules, dermatomyositis, leukemic infiltrates, and insulin lipodystrophy.

There is no effective therapy for this disease, not even corticosteroids. Occasionally sulfapyridine and chloroquine have seemed efficacious but iodides may cause an exacerbation of the eruption.

LIPOGRANULOMATOSIS OF ROTHMANN-MAKAI

This disorder is a form of circumscribed panniculitis, presenting as a relatively few subcutaneous nodules and plaques occurring on the lower extremities and trunk, occasionally on the arms and face. The lesions are firm or elastic and often are mildly tender on pressure. The overlying skin may be either hyperemic or normal. The nodules may disappear after a few days or weeks but usually persist for 6 to 12 months. The majority of cases occur in children and there are no systemic symptoms. No effective treatment is available. Histologically lipogranulomatosis resembles Weber-Christian disease so closely as to make differentiation often impossible. However, clinically the lack of fever and other systemic symptoms in Rothmann-Makai syndrome and the fact that the lesions do not occur in crops, all of which are prominent in Weber-Christian, distinguish the two conditions.

SUBCUTANEOUS FAT NECROSIS ASSOCIATED WITH PANCREATIC DISEASES

Although there had been rare reports of nodular subcutaneous fat necrosis in relation to pancreatitis since 1889, Szymanski and Bluefarb[19] in 1961 first clearly delineated the entity and pointed out the diagnostic histologic changes found on biopsy. They reported five cases, four with acute hemorrhagic pancreatitis and one with adenocarcinoma of the pancreas, in whom raised erythematous nodules (1 or 2 cm.) of the legs occurred. In two of the cases, the cutaneous lesions preceded the onset of abdominal symptoms.

Clinically, the nodules were not diagnostic and simulated either erythema nodosum, allergic vasculitis or a drug eruption. However, the histologic picture was characteristic. Except for an extension of the inflammatory reaction upward from the subcutis, there is usually no involvement of the epidermis or dermis. In the subcutis, foci of fat necrosis with "ghost cells" having thick "shadowy" walls and no nuclei, basophilic granular material representing calcium deposits, a wide variety of acute and chronic inflammatory cells around the necrotic areas and some hemorrhage are seen. This histologic picture does not occur in any other disease of the cutaneous fat tissue.

The authors postulate that trypsin liberated from the inflamed pancreas alters the vessel walls. Circulating lipase then leaks into the tissues and produces the fat necrosis and nodules. An elevated serum amylase was present in four cases. Serum lipases were not determined.

Recently Schrier and coworkers reviewed the 13 reported cases of subcutaneous fat necrosis in association with pancreatitis.[20] The lesions usually occurred on the legs, but on occasion appeared on the abdomen, chest, buttocks, and arms. The nodules were red, raised, and tender, persisted for days or a few weeks, and then regressed without

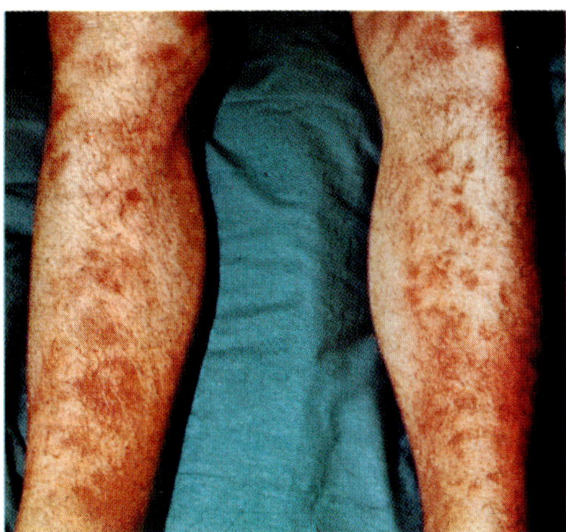

Fig. 7-7. Subcutaneous fat necrosis associated with pancreatitis. (Photo, courtesy Dr. L. F. Fenster.)

scarring (Fig. 7-7). The authors stated that the pathogenesis of the lesions was not clear. Though it was thought that circulating lipase was responsible, the serum lipase determination performed in their case gave a normal value.

DISCUSSION

As mentioned in the initial paragraph of this section, the nodose lesions of the legs do not readily lend themselves to a logical classification and therefore, we have simply listed and discussed them one by one. Attempts have been made to classify the various entities but the criteria employed, whether clinical or histologic, have not met with universal acceptance. Some authors have championed the distinctive nature of each disorder while others have maintained that such divisions are artificial and misleading.

Recently Fine and Meltzer[21] have presented the view that erythema nodosum, subacute nodular migratory panniculitis, nodular vasculitis and even erythema induratum do not differ significantly enough clinically, histologically or in response to therapy to warrant their separation into distinct entities. These authors prefer to group them under the term "chronic erythema nodosum," in which the major histologic finding is a septitis secondary to vasculitis. They do separate as distinct entities the primary panniculitides such as Weber-Christian disease, lipogranulomatosis of Rothmann and Makai and subcutaneous fat necrosis in pancreatic disease, since their histology is that of primary fat necrosis.

Whether such drastic grouping into two categories is correct or is as artificial as having too many disease entities must await further study and elucidation.

References

1. Michelson, H. E.: Inflammatory nodose lesions of the lower leg. Arch. Derm. Syph., *66*:327, 1952.

2. *Ibid.*

3. Editorial: "Nodules-on-the-leg" syndrome. New Eng. J. Med., *274*:463, 1966.

4. Holcomb, F. D.: Erythema nodosum associated with the use of an oral contraceptive: report of a case. Obstet. Gynec., *25*:156, Feb., 1965.

5. Baden, H. P., and Holcomb, F. D.: Erythema nodosum from oral contraceptives. Arch. Derm., *98*:634, July, 1968.

6. *Ibid.*

7. Lever, W. F.: Histopathology of the Skin. pp. 117-118, Philadelphia, J. B. Lippincott, 1961.

8. Feiwel, M., and Munro, D. D.: Diagnosis and treatment of erythema induratum (Bazin). Brit. Med. J., *1*:1109, Apr. 24, 1965.

9. Irgang, S.: Nodose erythema induratum (Bazin's disease). N. Y. State J. Med., *64*:2580, 1964.

10. Sandberg, D. H., and Adams, J. M.: Erythema induratum and streptococcosis. J. Ped., *61*:880, 1962.

11. Pillsbury, D. M., Shelley, W. B., and Kligman, A. M.: Dermatology. p. 527. Philadelphia, W. B. Saunders, 1956.

12. Feiwel, M., and Munro, D. D.: Diagnosis and treatment of erythema induratum (Bazin). Brit. Med. J., *1*:1109, Apr. 24, 1965.

13. Lever, W. F.: Histopathology of the Skin. pp. 231-234. Philadelphia, J. B. Lippincott, 1961.

14. Feiwel, M., and Munro, D. D.: Diagnosis and treatment of erythema induratum (Bazin). Brit. Med. J., *1*:1109, Apr. 24, 1965.

15. Montgomery, H., O'Leary, P.A., and Barker, N.W.: Nodular vascular disease of the legs: erythema induratum and allied conditions. JAMA., *128*:335, 1945.

16. Stringa, S.G., Bianchi, C., and Zingale, S.B.: Nodular vasculitis: immunofluorescent study. 7S gamma-globulin and complement (Blc-globulin) in lesions of nodular vasculitis, J. Invest. Derm., *46*:1, 1966.

17. Perry, H. O., and Winkelmann, R. K.: Subacute nodular migratory panniculitis. Arch. Derm., *89*:170, 1964.

18. *Ibid.*

19. Szymanski, F. J., and Bluefarb, S. M.: Nodular fat necrosis and pancreatic diseases. Arch. Derm., *83*:224, 1961.

20. Schrier, R. W., Melmon, K. L., and Fenster, L. F.: Subcutaneous nodular fat necrosis in pancreatitis. Arch. Intern. Med., *116*:832, 1965.

21. Fine, R. M., and Meltzer, H. D.: Chronic erythema nodosum. Arch. Derm., *100*:33, July, 1969.

8

Ulcers

Although the vast majority of ulcers of the leg are related to venous insufficiency, nonetheless one must always consider the possibility of other etiologic mechanisms. This is particularly true because differing etiologic factors may produce similar morphologic changes. For our purposes, the classification according to causal mechanism (Table 8-1) is relatively simple and reasonably complete.

Table 8-1

Classification of Ulcers of the Leg According to Causal Mechanism

- I. External
    - A. Primary
        - 1. Trauma
        - 2. Decubitus (trophic) ulcers
        - 3. Neurotic excoriations; factitious
    - B. Secondary to a Predisposing Lesion
        - 1. Burns (thermal and chemical)
        - 2. Radiodermatitis
        - 3. Neoplasms
- II. Internal
    - A. Vascular Diseases
        - 1. Arterial
            - a) Arteriosclerotic
            - b) Hypertensive ischemic
            - c) Thromboangiitis obliterans
            - d) Livedo reticularis
        - 2. Venous
            - a) Stasis
            - b) Thrombophlebitis
    - B. Blood Dyscrasias
        - 1. Anemias (heritable)
            - a) Sickle cell
            - b) Thalassemia
            - c) Congenital hemolytic
        - 2. Dysproteinemia
            - a) Macroglobulinemia
            - b) Cryoglobulinemia
    - C. Metabolic
        - 1. Diabetes mellitus
        - 2. Gout
    - D. Autoimmune Diseases
        - 1. Necrotizing angiitides
        - 2. Lupus erythematosus
        - 3. Scleroderma
        - 4. Rheumatoid arthritis
        - 5. Polyarteritis nodosa
        - 6. Pyoderma gangrenosum
    - E. Granulomas
        - 1. Microbiological
            - a) Syphilis
            - b) Erythema induratum
            - c) Atypical mycobacterial
            - d) Leprosy
            - e) Deep fungal infections
        - 2. Drugs
            - a) Halides
- III. Miscellaneous
    - A. Acrodermatitis chronica atrophicans
    - B. Atrophie blanche

EXTERNAL CAUSES

Ulcers produced by external causes are self-explanatory; diagnosis depends on the history. Examples of these not uncommon ulcers are presented in Figures 8-1, 8-2, 8-3, 8-4, 8-5, 8-6, 8-7.

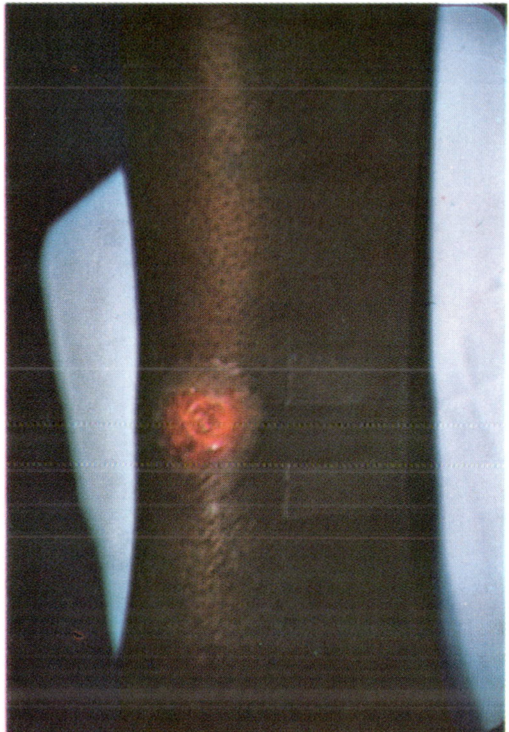

Fig. 8-1. Ulcer as a result of trauma.

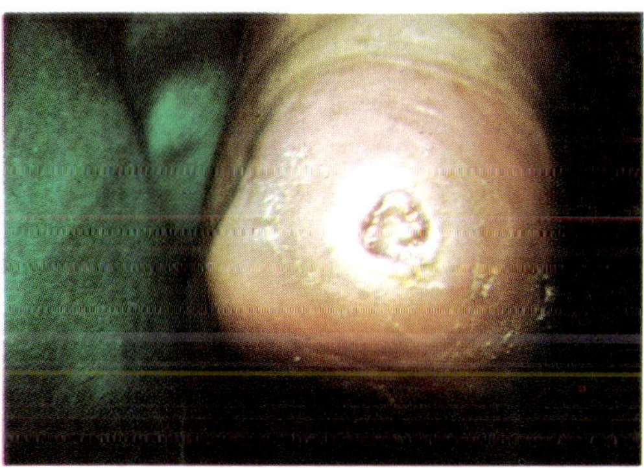

Fig. 8-2. Ulcer on heel resulting from shoe trauma.

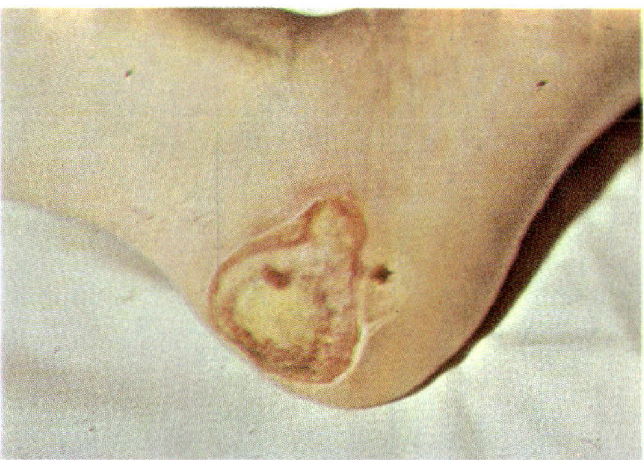

Fig. 8-3. Ulcer caused by pressure from brace.

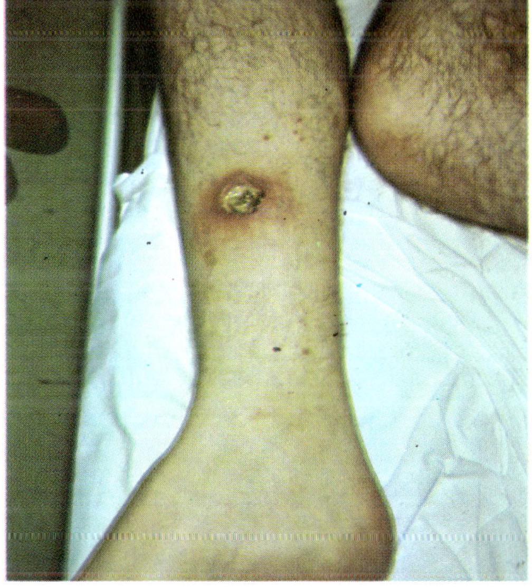

Fig. 8-4. Factitious ulcer. Patient applied cork soaked in phenol.

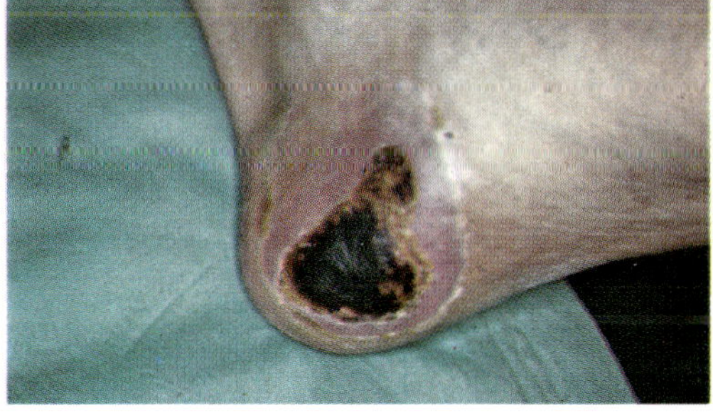

Fig. 8-5. Eschar adherent to ulcer secondary to third-degree burn from hot water bag.

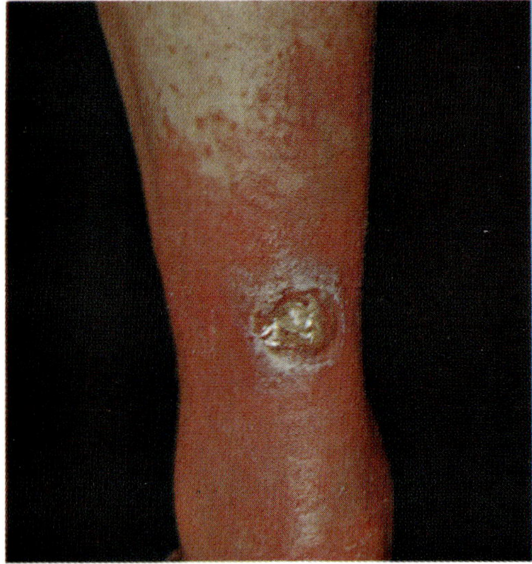

Fig. 8-6. Ulcer following x-ray treatment for epithelioma.

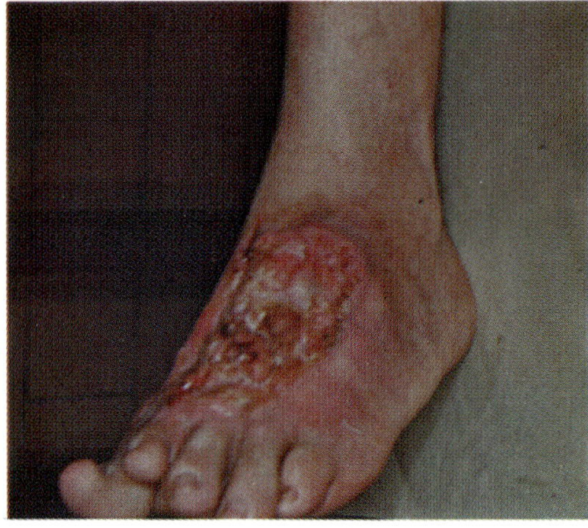

Fig. 8-7. Ulceration in squamous cell carcinoma.

INTERNAL CAUSES

It is not intended to present this group as final; a degree of overlapping is apparent, particularly in the category of the autoimmune diseases. This group has been discussed under vasculitis. Our attention will be directed toward the following selected ulcer syndromes.

Arteriosclerosis Obliterans (Figs. 8-8, 8-9). Leg ulcers of arteriosclerosis are due to infarction following the occlusion of an end artery. Arteriosclerotic ulcers tend to occur on the most distal portions of the extremity and thus are most often seen on the toes or feet. When an ischemic ulcer develops on the leg, it is almost invariably initiated by local trauma (i.e., the patient sustains a break in the skin which does not heal).

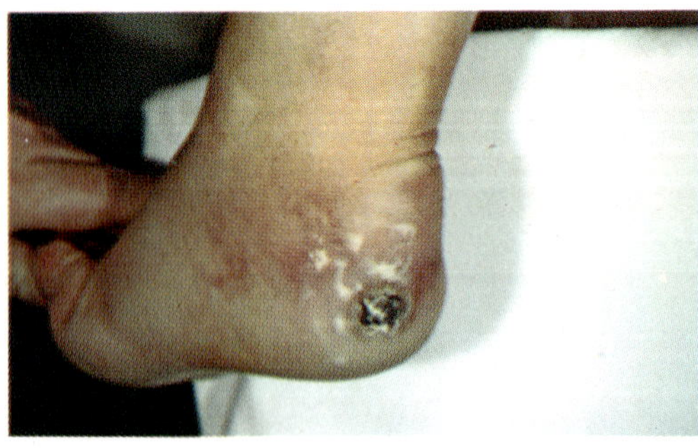

Fig. 8-8. Arteriosclerotic ulcer. Base of the ulcer is necrotic and hemorrhagic (infarcted tissue).

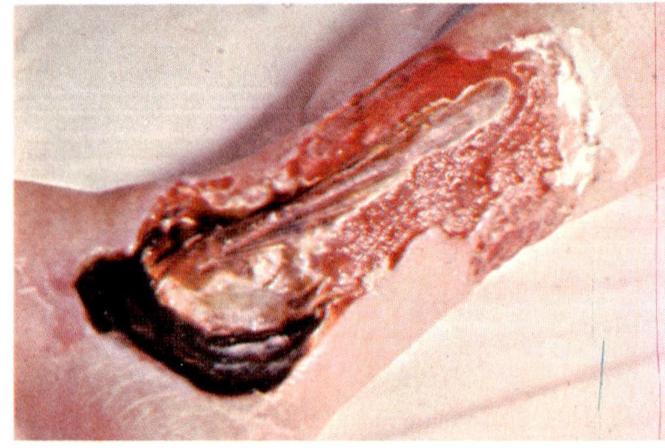

Fig. 8-9. Extensive ulceration in patient with arteriosclerosis and diabetes.

Since episodes of trauma may occur anywhere on the leg, there is no typical location for an ischemic ulcer, though many are located on the anterior portion of the limb because injuries are somewhat more common in that area. The base of the ulcer of arteriosclerosis obliterans is necrotic and hemorrhagic with a slight serous discharge. The adjacent skin does not exhibit signs of congestion or stasis changes. Rather, the ulcers often are surrounded by normal-appearing skin or by a rim of blue or purple skin representing infarcted tissue. The ulcers are frequently painful, often severely so, unless diabetic neuropathy is present.

Pedal pulses are often absent, thereby providing confirmatory evidence of arterial disease; they are, however, present in up to 40 percent of cases.

Therapy must be individualized in each patient; however, there are some general instructions which are applicable. The patient should be warned to avoid physical injury from any source and extremes of temperature. Caution against hot water or ice bags, and against bathing in very hot or very cold water. Interdict the use of tobacco because of nicotine's vasoconstrictor effects. Improve peripheral circulation with vasodilator drugs. Whiskey, 1 or 2 ounces, 4 times daily can also be effective as a mild vasodilator.

If the ulcer results from localized occlusion of small arterial branches, then some will heal solely from bed rest with elevation of the *head* of the bed and cool saline compresses. Others will respond to lumbar sympathectomy combined with complete excision of the ulcer and its surrounding rim of infarcted tissue, followed by a split-thickness skin graft from the abdomen onto the deep fascia. Occasionally arterial bypass surgery may be warranted. It is of utmost importance to determine that the arterial inflow at the iliac level is adequate before attempting reconstructive arterial surgery on the femoral-popliteal system.

Weismann and Johnson[1] reported the results of therapy in 31 cases of arteriosclerotic ulcers of the leg. Two healed on conservative therapy alone; the remaining 29 patients had a combination of medical and surgical treatment (20 improved and 5 eventually required amputation).

Hypertensive Ulcers of the Leg. These lesions usually occur in women between the ages of 50 and 70 who have been hypertensive for variable, but usually prolonged, periods.[2] A spontaneously occurring painful red plaque is the initial lesion, most commonly found on the lateral aspect of the ankle, though it may appear low on the posterior and lateral portions of the leg. Within 7 to 10 days, the plaque becomes blue and purpuric. An alternative initial lesion is a simple area of bluish purpuric discoloration of the skin. Soon a hemorrhagic bleb forms on the initial lesion, then breaks down and forms an ulcer which is pale, with little or no granulation tissue, and is very painful. A thick eschar often eventually forms over the ulcer. Generally the lesion develops slowly over a period of months. Some investigators report that the ulcers heal spontaneously in 6 to 9 months if irritating topical

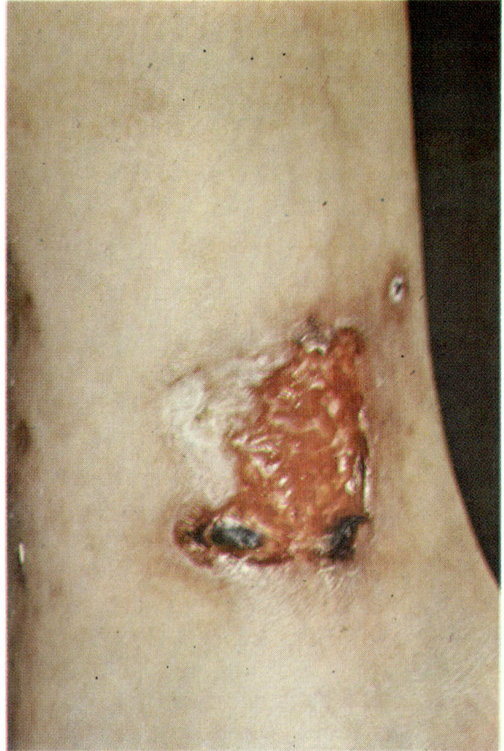

Fig. 8-10. Hypertensive ulcer in 52-year-old woman with 20-year history of hypertension.

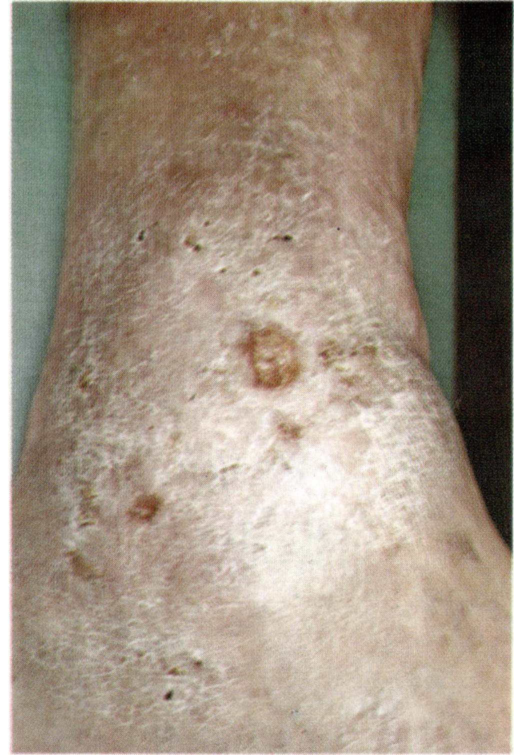

Fig. 8-11. Stasis ulcer. Characteristic localization: "spat" area.

medicaments are not applied; in our own and others' experience these ulcers tend to be extremely chronic and recalcitrant (Fig. 8-10).

Ulcerations in Thromboangiitis Obliterans. Thromboangiitis obliterans or Buerger's disease is a chronic inflammatory disease of the blood vessels with involvement of both arteries and veins occurring in males, particularly Jewish, between 20 to 40 years of age. Recurrent episodes of phlebitis and cellulitis occur and pain is a prominent symptom. Thrombosis of vessels leads to gangrene, necrosis and ulceration of the skin of the lower leg and foot.

Therapy is difficult. Tobacco and caffeine, mechanical and thermal (especially cold) trauma are to be avoided. Sympathectomy and other surgery, including amputation, are often required.

Ulcerations in Livedo Reticularis. Ulcers occasionally occur in areas of skin involved by livedo reticularis. (See Chap. 3 for further discussion.)

Stasis Ulcer. The deep venous system of the leg is separated from the superficial veins by the deep fascial layer. This structure provides good support to the deep veins. By contrast, the superficial veins are poorly supported by the subcutaneous tissue and skin. Numerous communicating veins, called perforators, connect the superficial veins to the deep system. The deep venous system contains valves to prevent backflow of blood and to facilitate venous return in a cephalad direction. Venous hypertension develops in the veins of the lower legs, resulting in chronic congestion of the tissues. If the perforating veins become incompetent, the pressure in the deep venous system is transmitted directly to the superficial veins.

The medial portions of the ankle and lower leg are the most common sites of stasis ulcers because it is there that the larger perforators occur in greatest numbers (Fig. 8-11).[3] Skin changes resulting from the chronic congestion are edema, pigmentation, induration and ulceration, eczematoid dermatitis, and subacute cellulitis. Often the origin of the ulcer is minor trauma, infection or occasionally the injudicious use of irritating topical medications.[4] Most ulcers caused by chronic venous insufficiency are rather shallow with irregularly shaped shelving edges, a reddish base with prominent granulation tissue, and surrounded by the mottled pigmentation of chronic stasis dermatitis. Some patients complain of pain or discomfort in the area of the ulcer, but severe pain is not associated with uncomplicated stasis ulcer.

The mainstays of therapy consist of bed rest, elevation of the legs (in severe chronic venous insufficiency, elevating the leg to at least 45° is absolutely essential), saline or dilute Burow's compresses and pressure gradient stockings.[5] Other therapeutic measures which may facilitate healing in selected cases are discussed at the end of the chapter.

Thrombophlebitic Ulcer. In contrast to a varicose ulcer, a post-thrombotic ulcer always penetrates the deep fascia. The edges of the ulcer are deep and indurated; the floor is covered with a thick, greyish, firmly adherent crust. Usually the surrounding skin is extensively indurated (Fig. 8-12) and pain is a constant accompaniment.

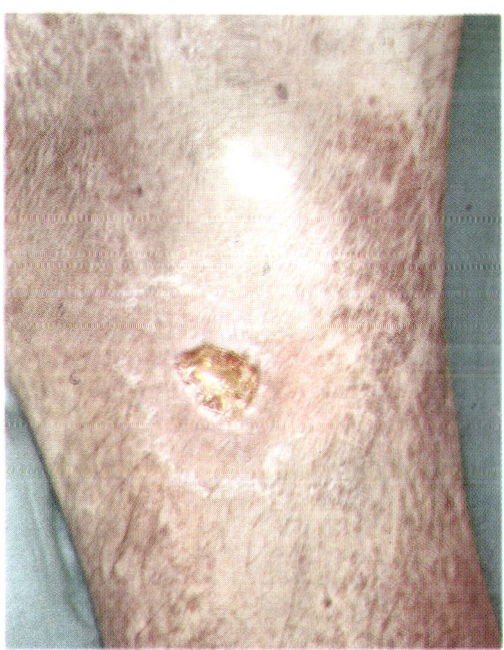

Fig. 8-12. Thrombophlebitic ulcer penetrating to deep fascia.

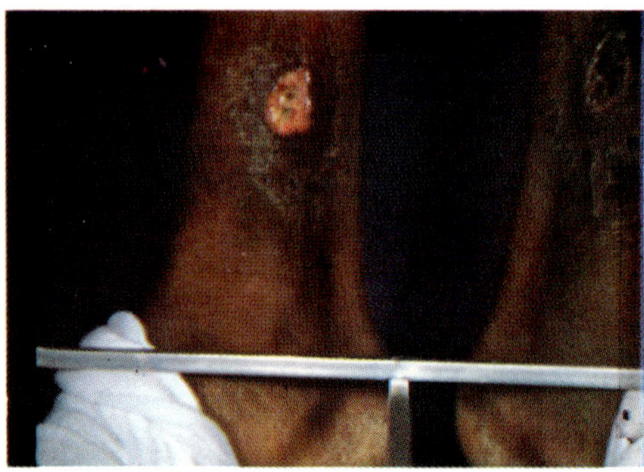

Fig. 8-13. Ulcers with sickle cell anemia.

Sickle Cell Anemia. Many patients with sickle cell disease who survive into adolescence or adulthood have chronic leg ulcers or the scars of previous ulcers. These ulcerations may antedate other clinical manifestations of sickle cell disease. The leg lesions themselves (Fig. 8-13) are not distinctive enough to permit a diagnosis clinically, but the ulcer may be the chief complaint and lead to the detection of sickle cell anemia. The diagnosis is confirmed by laboratory studies showing a normocytic and normochromic anemia with sickling of cells, and by hemoglobin electrophoresis.

Ulcers Associated With Thalassemia. Leg ulcers occur rarely in Mediterranean anemia, only 10 cases having been reported in American literature. The ulcers occur around the ankle, may be either unilateral or bilateral, and involve both the medial and lateral malleolar areas (Fig. 8-14). Leg ulcers appear only in patients with thalassemia minor, since only a rare patient with thalassemia major survives beyond puberty. The pathogenesis of the ulcers is not known. Samitz *et al.*[6] postulated that the etiologic factors giving rise to the ulcers were multiple and nonspecific: trauma, infection, excoriation, hypoxia from chronic anemia, and peripheral slowing of blood flow. Therapy should be conservative; the ulcers have healed with the application of soaks, rest, elevation, debridement, grafts, Ace bandages, and Unna's boots. Transfusions and splenectomy have not proved beneficial to the healing of the ulcers.

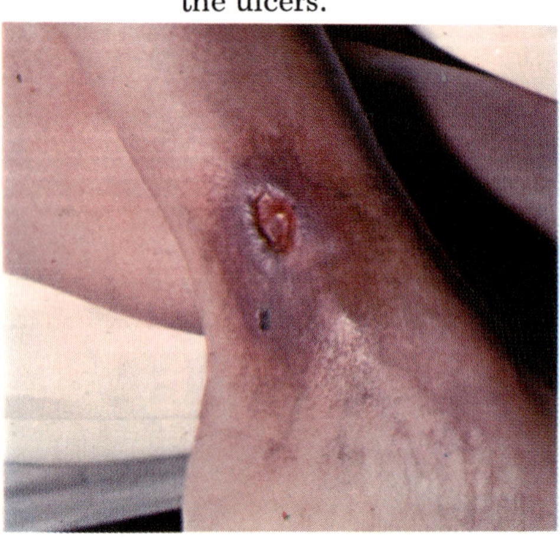

Fig. 8-14. Ulcer in thalassemia.

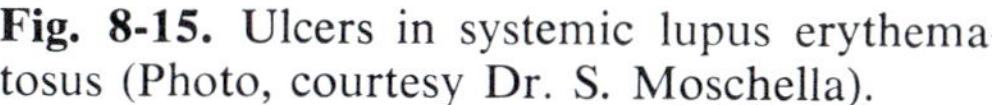

Fig. 8-15. Ulcers in systemic lupus erythematosus (Photo, courtesy Dr. S. Moschella).

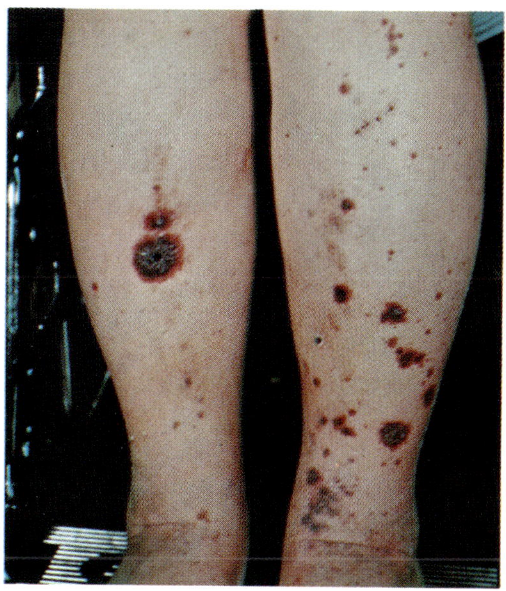

Systemic Lupus Erythematosus. Although leg ulcers have been reported in lupus erythematosus on several occasions, they do not occur commonly in the disease. Tuffanelli and Dubois[7] noted leg ulcers in 5.6 percent of their series of 520 cases. The ulcers usually occurred over the pretibial or malleolar areas (Fig. 8-15), ranged in diameter from 1 to 10 cm. and had smooth, erythematous borders. The ulcers may be associated with livedo reticularis or cryoglobulinemia. Laboratory tests that may be helpful include those used in diagnosing systemic lupus erythematosus, skin biopsy and immunofluorescent studies. Vasculitis of medium-sized vessels resulting in infarction of the skin and subcutaneous tissues is presumably the cause of the ulceration. Leg ulcers in association with systemic lupus erythematosus heal rapidly on steroid therapy, whereas traumatic ulcers occurring in areas of atrophy heal slowly.

Sclerodermatous Leg Ulcers. In systemic sclerosis, ulcerations of the distal portions of the extremities as well as over the joints[8] are common. On the legs, the ulcers usually occur over the knees and ankles. The lesion may be a shallow erosion or a deep indolent ulceration with deposits of calcium in the crater. The ulcer itself may suggest the diagnosis of scleroderma, but the diagnosis is usually made by the cutaneous changes elsewhere and by biopsy.

These ulcers are notoriously recalcitrant to therapy. Herman *et al.*[9] reported one case in which skin grafting was successful. Early reports suggested that DMSO might prove efficacious in healing these troublesome lesions; however, further studies are necessary to substantiate this finding.

Ulcers Associated With Rheumatoid Arthritis. Vasculitis may occur in rheumatoid arthritis and result in a wide spectrum of lesions, ranging

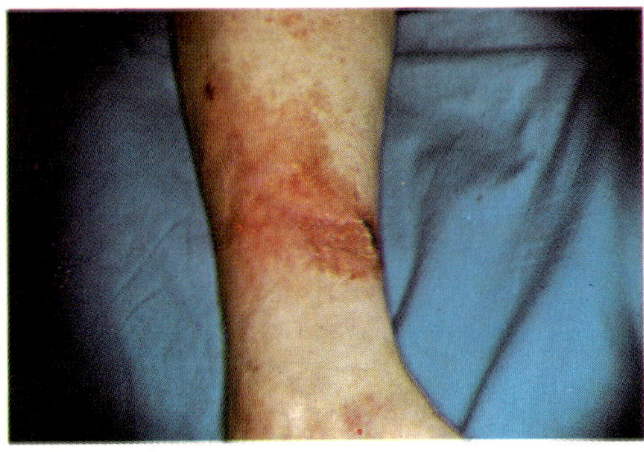

Fig. 8-16. Ulcer complicating rheumatoid arthritis.

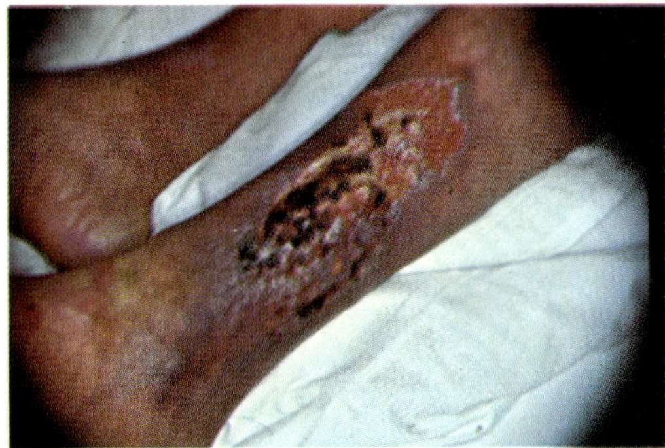

Fig. 8-17. Ulceration in necrotizing vasculitis.

from ischemic skin changes to widespread fatal systemic involvement. There is some evidence that the vasculitis is occasionally related to prolonged corticosteroid therapy or its abrupt cessation.[10] The skin manifestations of the vasculitis seen in rheumatoid arthritis may consist of purpura, gangrene, necrosis of subcutaneous nodules or ulcerations (Fig. 8-16).

In a series of approximately 2000 cases of rheumatoid arthritis, 12 patients had ulcerations of the skin, primarily located on the lower leg. Among 128 cases of rheumatoid arthritis hospitalized at the New Orleans V.A. Hospital, 5 had ischemic skin lesions of the extremities.[11]

Ischemic skin lesions, including ulcers, tend to occur in the patient who has severe rheumatoid arthritis, associated subcutaneous nodules, and a high titer of rheumatoid factor in his serum. This combination of clinical features has been suggested as a relative contraindication to steroid therapy. It also has been suggested that avoidance of (1) high doses of corticosteroids, (2) fluctuations in dosage, and (3) abrupt withdrawal of steroids might prevent the appearance of these ischemic lesions.

Ulcers in Other Autoimmune Diseases. The ulcers seen in association with the necrotizing angiitides (Figs. 8-17), polyarteritis nodosa, and pyoderma gangrenosum have been discussed in the section on page 79.

Granulomatous Ulcers of the Leg. The ulcerations which may occur on the leg in late syphilis (gummas) (Figs. 8-18, 8-19), erythema induratum, atypical mycobacterial infections, leprosy, and deep fungal infections (Fig. 8-20) may frequently be misdiagnosed because the correct etiologic possibility is simply not considered. Any ulceration which is clinically atypical, or does not heal under conservative therapy, should be biopsied and appropriate stains performed to ascertain whether one of the above causes is present and to rule out the possibility that the ulcer represents an indolent malignancy. Additional studies, such as bacterial and fungal cultures and serologic tests for syphilis, also may be indicated.

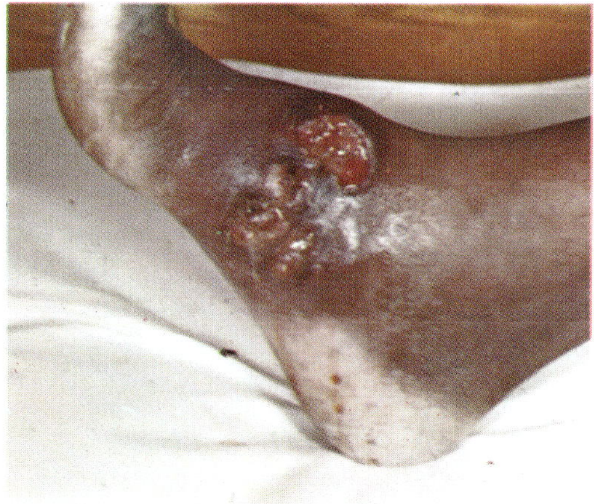

Fig. 8-18. Ulcerative gummas.

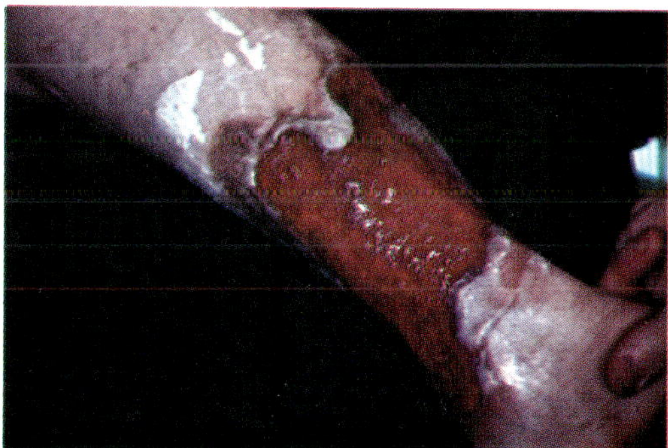

Fig. 8-19. Ulcerative gumma.

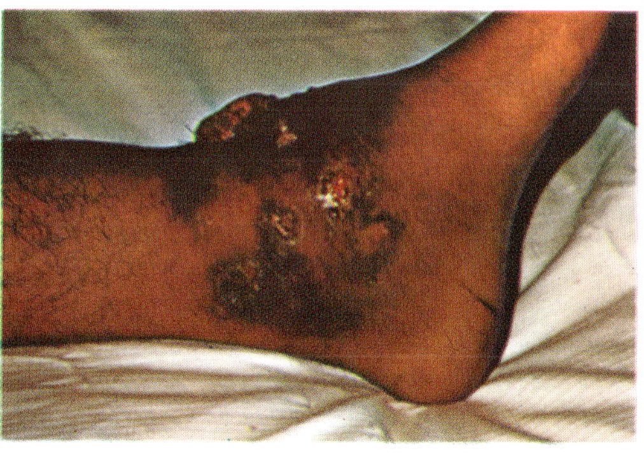

Fig. 8-20. Ulcers in maduromycosis.

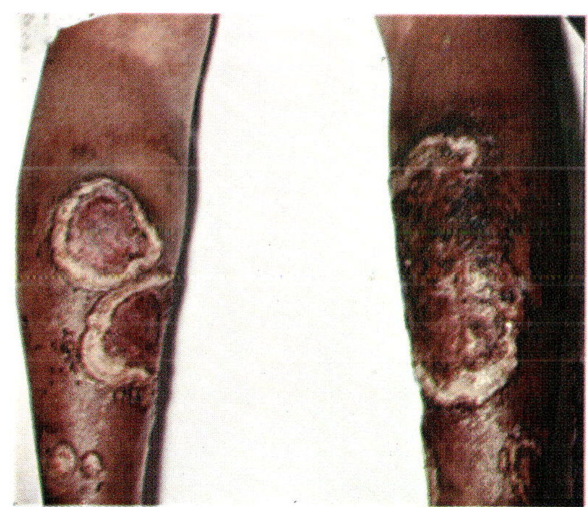

Fig. 8-21. Ulcers in granulomas of bromoderma.

Ulcerations Due to Halides. Both bromide and iodide compounds may produce a wide variety of skin eruptions. The most common dermatosis is an acneform or follicular pustular eruption. However, granulomatous fungating or ulcerative lesions of the extremities (Fig. 8-21) also are seen; this possibility must be considered in the diagnosis of ulcers that do not respond to the usual modes of therapy, particularly if they have a granulomatous border. Though most drug eruptions fade within two weeks after withdrawal of the offending agent, the lesions produced by the halides characteristically are slow to involute.

DIAGNOSTIC APPROACH TO LEG ULCERS

In the evaluation of a patient with leg ulcers a careful systematic approach is essential to ensure the greatest probability of arriving at an etiologic diagnosis. The first two steps in this approach are the most important: (1) a careful history; and (2) a complete physical examination.

Following the completion of these steps a variety of tests may be utilized to establish the diagnosis. In some patients only one or two tests may be necessary while in others a wide spectrum of studies is essential. Among the procedures indicated are:

1. Complete blood count
2. Blood chemistry profile
3. Serologic test for syphilis
4. Urinalysis
5. Skin biopsy
6. Bacterial smear, anaerobic and aerobic cultures
7. Chest x-ray
8. Fungal KOH preparation and culture, including special culture media when indicated
9. Tuberculin and fungal skin tests
10. Serum and/or immune electrophoresis
11. LE cell prep, latex fixation, sickle cell prep and hemoglobin electrophoresis
12. Bone marrow or lymph node biopsy

Additional x-ray, fluorescent antibody and immunoglobulin studies and other systemic evaluations may also be indicated in specific cases.

A point worth stressing is that a biopsy should be done in any ulcer which is atypical in appearance, or which does not respond to therapy; in this way unsuspected vasculitis, malignancy or granulomatous infections may be discovered.

Treatment

Hosts of topical preparations have been recommended for local therapy and this itself suggests that none is entirely satisfactory. Furthermore, one should always keep in mind the possibility of adverse reactions caused by some of these preparations. Topical antibacterial agents and antibiotics, such as Furacin and neomycin, are common offenders. Occasionally the preservative used in the ointment is responsible. We have observed several cases in which the preservatives, paraben and ethylenediamine, have aggravated eczematization because of sensitization. It is therefore advisable to avoid many of these preparations. In fact, it is a good general rule to avoid any type of ointment, especially on ischemic ulcers. Simple, bland applications are the measures of choice.

For local infection: In a recent study on the bacterial flora of peripheral vascular ulcers, Friedman and Gladstone[12] were unable to show whether the surface infection found in clinically inflamed ulcers is significant and warrants antibacterial therapy. In ulcers infected with Pseudomonas, Calloway[13] has reported on the use of ¼ to ½ percent acetic acid. In our experience we have found this highly effective.

Enzymatic debridement is useful to clean away detritus but does not otherwise contribute to healing of the ulcer and should be discontinued when the ulcer is clean. The most commonly used are Biozyme, Varidase, Chymar, Elase and Tryptar. A combination of papain and urea (Panafil) is also useful for enzymatic debridement.

Whole blood or powdered blood cells have been advocated to stimulate healing of both ischemic and stasis ulcers when applied to the ulcer surface. We prefer packing the ulcer with Gelfoam powder for 24 hours followed by cleansing with fresh hydrogen peroxide. The application of the powder is repeated, and the treated area covered with a pressure bandage. This regimen can be carried out once a day by the patient himself.

Occlusive agents such as gold leaf, aluminum foil and polyethylene film have been advanced to promote healing and reepithelization. Smith *et al.*,[14] in a partially controlled study, reported that the response rate (percentage reepithelization per day) of ulcers treated with gold leaf was no better than the response rate of those treated with a simple dressing. In our experience, aluminum foil has proved helpful in selected cases. We prefer thin aluminum foil. It is inexpensive, readily available and much easier to apply than gold leaf. The patient can carry out the treatment once a day and be followed at intervals of one or two weeks. We emphasize that the foil should be cut to measure approximately 1 mm. less than the size of the ulcer. The metal is held in place by covering with a gauze pad or an eye pad dressing.

Occasionally reepithelization of an ulcer may be retarded because of excess granulation tissue. Pressure with foam rubber pads, or the application of silver nitrate 0.5 percent are effective in controlling the problem.

Ambulatory therapy of resistant leg ulcers associated with venous disease and accompanied by persistent edema can be carried out by the use of an Unna's Boot.

The ulcer is cleansed with hydrogen peroxide, packed with Gelfoam powder and covered with a gauze pressure bandage. An Unna's Boot (Dome-Paste Bandage, Dome Laboratories) is then applied from the base of the toes to just below the knee with the pressure greatest at the ankles, progressively lessening as one ascends the leg to the knee and least at the base of the toes. Tubegauz and an elastic stocking or bandage may be worn over the Unna's Boot. The boot is changed every few days depending on the amount of serous drainage from the ulcer and the dermatitis. The Primer and Flexoplast combination (Edward Taylor, Ltd.), a modified Unna's Boot, has also proved effective.

Resistant venous ulcers which do not respond to conservative treatment can be treated by skin grafting on an outpatient basis.[15]

Bed rest is probably the most effective treatment for chronic leg ulceration. For hospitalized patients, topical oxygen therapy can be used to stimulate reepithelization in indolent ulcers. Elliott[16] described the following simple device: "The affected extremity is placed in a plastic bag and the open end is closed above the ulcer with a rubber band. Oxygen from a tank is allowed to flow through a plastic tube into the deflated bag until it is completely distended. Treatment should last 30 minutes 3 to 4 times daily." Specially constructed devices using hyperbaric oxygen were reported by Fischer[17] as a promising approach to the treatment of certain ulcerations unresponsive to other forms of treatment.

Internal medications, as a rule, have no merit in the management of stasis ulcers. Recently Husain[18] has reported good results in the healing of chronic leg ulcers with bed rest and topical therapy combined with the use of oral zinc sulfate. Presumably zinc accelerates wound healing. In his study, the zinc sulfate group of patients seemed clinically to show more rapid epithelization than the control group. The medication was given in capsules containing 220 mg. zinc sulfate three times daily, half an hour after meals. In a study by Halsted and Smith[19], the mean plasma-zinc in patients with indolent ulcers was significantly lower than controls. Upon treatment with zinc sulfate, the plasma-zinc level rose significantly, indicating good absorption. Much more data will be necessary to determine whether zinc sulfate is effective and what possible cumulative toxic effects it may carry with its use.

References

1. Weismann, R.E., and Johnson, M.: Ischemic ulcers of the leg. Surg. Clin. N. Am., *43*:1263, Oct., 1963.

2. Woolling, K.R.: Hypertensive-ischemic ulcer. JAMA, *187:* 196, 1964.

3. Hines, E.A., Jr.: The differential diagnosis of chronic ulcer of the leg. Circulation, *27*:989, 1963.

4. Lofgren, K.A.: Stasis ulcer. Mayo Clin. Proc., *40*:564, 1965.

5. Beninson, J.: Stasis dermatitis and leg ulcers. Postgrad. Med., *36*:524, 1964.

6. Samitz, M.H., Waldorf, D.S., and Shrager, J.: Leg ulcers in Mediterranean anemia. Arch. Derm., *90*:567, 1964.

7. Tuffanelli, D. L., and Dubois, E.L.: Cutaneous manifestations of systemic lupus erythematosus. Arch. Derm., *90*:377, 1964.

8. Leinwand, I., Duryee, A.W., and Richter, M.N.: Scleroderma (based on a study of over 150 cases). Ann Int. Med., *41*:1003, 1954.

9. Herman, B.E., *et al.*: Successful skin graft in patient with generalized scleroderma. JAMA, *182*:578, 1962.

10. Johnson, R.L., *et al.*: Steroid therapy and vascular lesions in rheumatoid arthritis. Arth. Rheum., *2*:224, 1959.

11. O'Quinn, S.E., Kennedy, C.B., and Baker, DeW. T.: Peripheral vascular lesions in rheumatoid arthritis. Arch. Derm., *92*:489, 1965.

12. Friedman, S.A., and Gladstone, J.L.: The bacterial flora of peripheral vascular ulcers. Arch. Derm. *100*:29, July, 1969.

13. Callaway, J.L.: Chronic leg ulcers. JAMA, *186*:1080, Dec., 1963.

14. Smith, K.W., Oden, P.W., and Blaylock, W.K.: A comparison of gold leaf and other occlusive therapy. Arch. Derm., *96*:703, Dec., 1967.

15. Chilvers, A.S., and Freeman, G.K.: Outpatient skin grafting of venous ulcers. Lancet, *2*:1087, Nov. 22, 1969.

16. Elliott, J.A.: Stasis dermatitis and stasis ulcer. *In* Howard F. Conn (ed.): Current Therapy. p. 505, Philadelphia, W.B. Saunders, 1967.

17. Fischer, B.H.: Topical hyperbaric oxygen treatment of pressure sores and skin ulcers. Lancet, *2*:405, Aug. 23, 1969.

18. Husain, S.L.: Oral zinc sulphate in leg ulcers, Lancet *1*:1069, May 31, 1969.

19. Halsted, J.A. and Smith, J.C., Jr.: Plasma-zinc in health and disease. Lancet, *1*:322, Feb. 14, 1970.

9

Immersion Injuries

WARM WATER IMMERSION FOOT*

The name warm water immersion injury refers to the syndrome which has the following signs and symptoms: whitening and wrinkling of the sole with associated pain and/or altered sensation of the sole.[1] The importance of the disorder lies in the fact that it is an occupational hazard among certain military combat elements operating in tropical areas although it can disable any susceptible individual who is exposed to the proper environmental conditions.

There is some confusion regarding the relationship between immersion foot and warm water immersion injury. From a practical standpoint the etiologic factors that cause both these conditions are identical except for the element of cold. Both disorders develop as a result of prolonged immersion in a wet environment. Thus, both might be more properly classified under the descriptive term "immersion injury." As classically described, immersion foot occurs when the water temperature is between 32° and 60° F. and is capable of producing permanent tissue damage. On the other hand, warm water immersion injury occurs after prolonged exposure to water warmer than 60° F. and is known to cause only temporary disability. It should be pointed out that the figure of 60° F. is an arbitrary one; there is no exact temperature level at which one suddenly develops one disorder or the other.[2]

The initial signs of warm water immersion injury occur during the first 24 hours when the weight-bearing surfaces of the sole begin to wrinkle and turn white. More often than not the skin covering the lateral and dorsal aspects of the foot develops fine wrinkles and some whitening as the feet continue to be exposed to the wet environment. Within 48 to 72 hours the individual develops symptoms related to the weight-bearing surfaces, especially under the metatarsal areas. These symptoms are variously described as burning pain, pinching, tingling, itching and pain or aching on bearing weight. It is at this point that the individual becomes a victim of warm water immersion injury and during combat he becomes a casualty who requires evacuation from the battlefield.

There is a wide range of susceptibility to the effects of occluded wet environment. Many individuals develop varying degrees of whitening and wrinkling but no symptoms, and there are a few individuals who show almost no evidence of immersion injury even after several days in water. On occasion, one notes a marked inexplicable difference be-

*In collaboration with G. T. Anderson, M.D.

tween the feet in the same individual. The areas of the sole with thickened stratum corneum are the first areas to develop signs of immersion injury and persons with thick calluses are generally those individuals who develop symptoms more quickly and to a greater degree (Figs. 9-1, 9-2). The wrinkling of the sole frequently becomes so marked that deep fissure-like grooves appear on the sole in the areas between the metatarsal heads. Severe maceration generally develops between and under all toes.

The clinical course during the postimmersion period appears directly related to the severity of the immersion injury. In those individuals who have been affected to a lesser degree, one notes that the soles have nearly regained their preimmersion appearance within 24 hours. In the moderately severe cases, one notes a mild erythema, tenderness on bearing weight and slight edema of the weight-bearing surfaces which generally disappears gradually over the first 24 to 36 hours. In the most severe cases, the symptoms and signs can take several days to disappear. As the injured stratum corneum begins to dry and exfoliate, fissures can appear beneath the toes and may be a source of secondary pyoderma.

The etiology of warm water immersion injury is not fully understood. The histology has never been reported. Clinical observations suggest, however, that the signs and symptoms of this condition are the result of the absorption of water by the stratum corneum and the edema of the underlying tissues. The absorption of water by the stratum corneum makes it thicker, opaque and white. Fibrous attachments of the sole to the underlying fascia probably help produce the convoluted and wrinkled appearance of the sole when edema appears. It seems likely that the symptom of pain, and possibly the edema, occur as the result of the simple traumatic experience of a thick water-laden wrinkled epidermis impinging upon the soft, sensitive tissues beneath.

The most effective prophylaxis for immersion injury is drying the feet for a period of 6 to 8 hours out of every 24, (e.g., sleeping without shoes). This had been shown experimentally[3] and has been known by military commanders for years. This fact possibly explains why this disorder has not been reported in people who do not wear occlusive footgear in a wet environment. The obvious treatment for warm water immersion injury is to maintain a condition of cleanliness and dryness until the skin over the feet has reverted to normal.

EROSION INJURY*

Another clinical expression of immersion injury has been noted during certain combat operations conducted over sandy, muddy terrain during periods of constant rain. This injury begins to appear in certain individuals within 24 hours as multiple, red, sharply circumscribed superficial erosions appearing much like the base of fresh bullae (Figs. 9-3, 9-4) and is generally seen independently of warm water immersion injury because the incubation period is much shorter. As the factor of time in a muddy, wet environment increases, one can see both condi-

*In collaboration with G. T. Anderson, M.D.

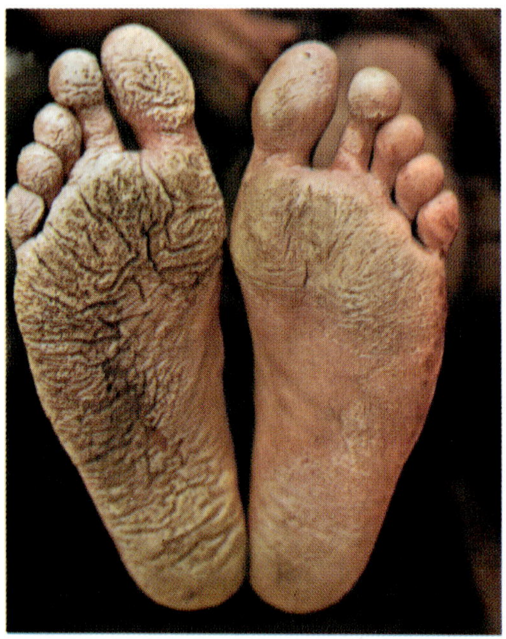

Fig. 9-1. Warm water immersion injury showing marked difference in response to the injury in one individual.

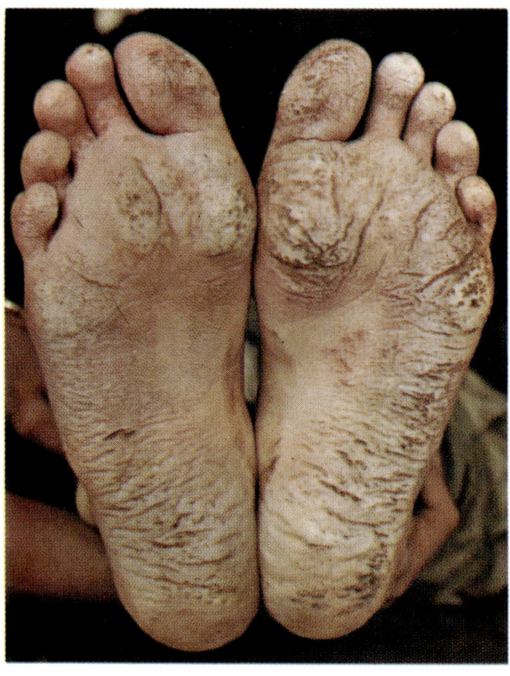

Fig. 9-2. Warm water immersion injury showing more severe response in calloused areas.

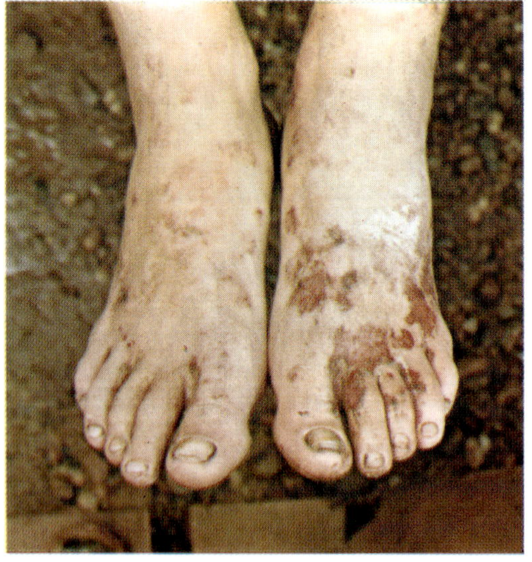

Fig. 9-3. Erosion injury.

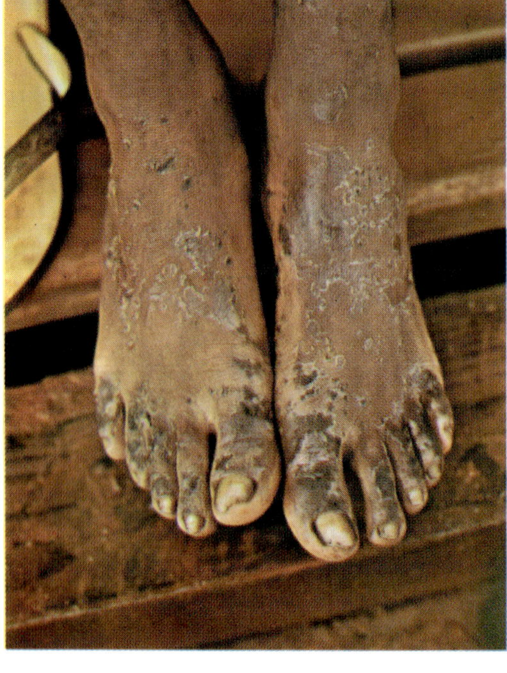

Fig. 9-4. Erosion injury 3 days postimmersion.

tions concurrently. There is a marked individual variation in the extent of this disorder from a few bright red patches on the dorsum of the toes to extensive erosions from boot top level to the soles. Burning pain is the presenting symptom and it frequently becomes so severe that the individual has to be evacuated from combat. All patients with this condition state that they can feel their skin being abraded by the dirt from the paddies and fine sand from the streams sifting into and through their boots. Fine particles of sand or dirt can usually be palpated on the surface of these lesions.

The developmental dynamics of erosion injury are not fully understood. Some medical officers have verbally reported that bullae are occasionally noted prior to the appearance of the erosion, but the author has never been witness to this fact. One thing is clinically apparent, walking for extended periods over sandy, wet or muddy terrain while wearing boots, with or without socks, is common to all cases.

After removal of the patient to a dry environment, the lesions of erosion injury form a thin, dry crust and the patient experiences healing in several days. As in warm water immersion injury, secondary pyoderma can occur during the postimmersion period and can obviously extend the period of disability.

PITTED KERATOLYSIS

For completeness in a discussion of warm water immersion foot injury one must also include a third entity, keratoma plantare sulcatum, which was first decribed in 1910 by Castellani.[4] Because of the recently intensified studies on the feet, it has become known as pitted keratolysis[5] and is commonly associated with warm water immersion foot injury. It may be seen frequently in patients who do not develop the full-blown syndrome.

Pitted keratolysis occurs in individuals under combat conditions, whose feet are continually wet for 3 days or more.[6] Small shallow pits develop in the stratum corneum of the sole over the weight-bearing surfaces, particularly the heels, balls of the feet and toe pads. The lesions begin to occur after 24 to 48 hours of immersion and range from 2 to 4 mm. in diameter and 1 to 2 mm. in depth. The number of pits ranges from 5 to more than 100. At times, individual lesions coalesce to form shallow pits 1 to 2 cm. in diameter. Some of the pits have a dirty brown to black pigmentation of the crater floor and walls which cannot be removed by washing. The lesions are asymptomatic and most are completely healed and the feet regain the preimmersion appearance 48 to 72 hours after the patient is removed from the wet environment. These findings occur more frequently in individuals with hyperhidrosis.

Biopsy of lesions reveals that the pits are confined to the stratum corneum.[7] The floor and walls contain an organism consisting of filamentous and coccal forms. The filaments are branched and are 1 to 2 microns in diameter and the coccal forms are 2 to 3 microns in diameter. An organism identified as corynebacterium species has been cultured from lesions of pitted keratolysis. The same organism has been used to produce pitted keratolysis in human subjects.

Recently, Lamberg[8] described symptomatic pitted keratolysis in which the usual asymptomatic pits are accompanied by plaques of reddened thinning and distinct tenderness on the soles occurring in areas of greatest pressure. Pain is sufficient to prevent walking and as much as 14 days of bed rest may be necessary before the patient can ambulate without pain.

Forty percent formalin in aquaphor has been effective in both the asymptomatic and symptomatic forms of pitted keratolysis.

References

1. Buckels, L.J., Gill, K.A., and Anderson, G.T.: Prophylaxis of warm-water-immersion foot. JAMA, *200*:681, 1967.

2. Taplin, D., and Zaias, N.: Tropical immersion foot syndrome. Military Medicine, *131*:814, Sept., 1966.

3. Taplin, D., Zaias, N., and Blank, H.: The role of temperature in tropical immersion foot syndrome. JAMA, *202*:546, 1967.

4. Castellani, A.: Keratoma plantare sulcatum. J. Ceylon Gr. Brit. Med. Assoc., *7*:10, 1910.

5. Zaias, N., Taplin, D., and Rebell, G.: Pitted keratolysis, Arch. Derm., *92*:151, 1965.

6. Gill, K.A., Jr., and Buckels, L.J.: Pitted keratolysis, Arch. Derm., *98*:7, 1968.

7. *Ibid.*

8. Lamberg, S.I.: Symptomatic pitted keratolysis, Arch. Derm., *100*:10, 1969.

10

Sweat Disorders

Many mammals possess eccrine sweat glands on their foot pads, presumably to moisten the skin surface and thereby improve their grip. Eccrine sweat glands are widely distributed, numerous and highly developed in some of the higher primates where they serve a thermoregulatory function. In man eccrine glands reach the maximum degree of development. They are located on all areas of the body surface except the lips and mucous membrane portion of the genitalia and are most concentrated on the soles, palms and in the axillae.

The first appearance of the forerunner of eccrine glands is a specialized downgrowth of the epidermis in the 4th fetal month. The sweat glands begin to develop first in the palms and soles and then elsewhere over the skin of the body. No additional sweat glands are formed after birth. Many sweat glands which are histologically normal are nonfunctioning. By 2½ years of age, all eccrine sweat glands which are to be functional in the adult have become active.

Thermal sweating is regulated by a hypothalamic center that responds to changes in the temperature of the blood perfusing it. This type of sweating is rather generalized, occurring most prominently on the upper trunk and face. The eccrine glands of the palms and soles respond only weakly to thermal stimuli.

Mental, emotional or psychic sweating is most striking on the palms and soles, and weaker responses from eccrine glands elsewhere. Centers for psychic sweating are located in the frontal region of the brain but the precise position and pathways are not known.

The eccrine sweat glands depend upon an intact sympathetic nerve supply to function. This sympathetic innervation is unusual in that it is cholinergic. Sweat is usually hypotonic and contains sodium, chloride, potassium, urea and lactate as its most significant constituents.

HYPERHIDROSIS

Hyperhidrosis is an abnormal increase in the amount of sweat produced; on the feet it may be part of a generalized hyperhidrosis, or it may be local.

Generalized hyperhidrosis may be due to such factors as a hot, humid environment, increased internal heat production by work or exercise, febrile illnesses, hypothalamic disorders or endocrine disorders.

Although hyperhidrosis of the feet is often due to emotional stimuli, there are also numerous individuals in whom there is no apparent primary emotional disorder. Rather, there would seem to exist some

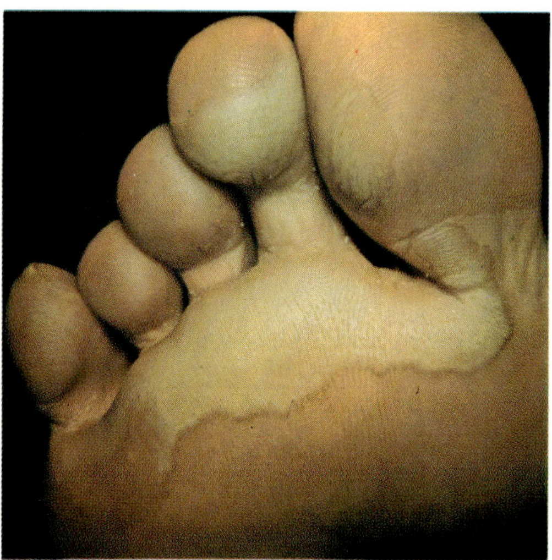

Fig. 10-1. Hyperhidrosis, undersurface of toes.

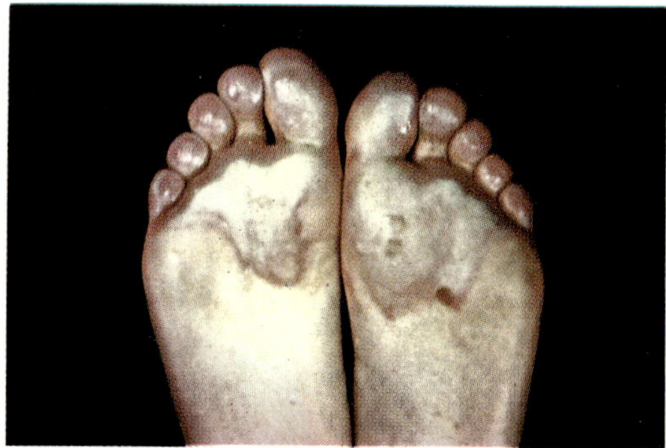

Fig. 10-2. Hyperhidrosis of soles.

facilitation of the neural pathways causing physiological psychic sweating. In these persons hyperhidrosis may be virtually constant. Other causes may be poor foot mechanics, faulty footwear, neural changes (neuritis, syringomyelia, tabes, paresis), and certain skin lesions (trench foot, frostbite).

In most cases of hyperhidrosis of the feet, moisture may be seen; however, in many instances the moisture can only be felt. The feet feel wet and soggy. The skin is whitish and may be macerated. Between the toes especially there is maceration and there may be splitting of the skin. The skin may be thickened and even appear worm-eaten (Figs. 10-1, 10-2). Either sex may be affected and the onset is usually in childhood or around puberty. The hyperhidrosis may persist for many years; however it tends to lessen spontaneously after the age of 25 years. The disorder may show a familial tendency.

Many of these cases may be mistaken for fungal infections. Hyperhidrosis may predispose and prepare a favorable soil for fungal infection. The paradox however is seen in children. Hyperhidrosis of the feet is particularly common in children; yet fungal infection is relatively rare before puberty. Hyperhidrosis may also be a predisposing factor for contact dermatitis and dyshidrotic eczema.

In an entity known as *symmetric lividity of the soles*, there is a hyperkeratotic reaction of the sole to hyperhidrosis. The condition is characterized by cyanotic color changes reflecting the vasomotor activity seen in association with hypersympathotonia and presents as bluish-red plaques of thickened, soggy hyperkeratosis (Fig. 10-3). The disorder is seen often in young foot soldiers.

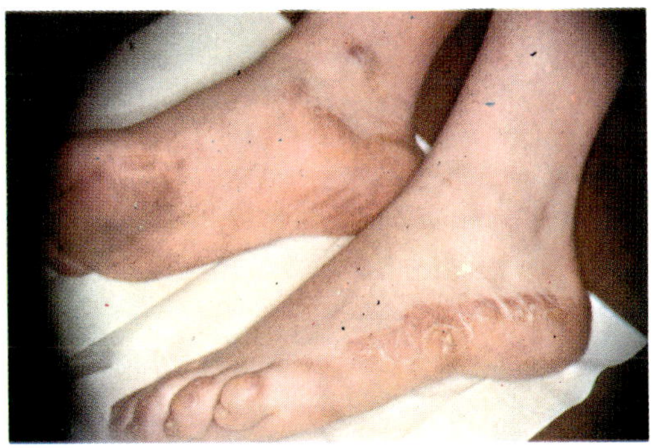

Fig. 10-3. Symmetric erythema of soles.

Treatment

Systemic and topical therapy are by no means satisfactory.

Systemic therapy with anticholinergic drugs (e.g., Pro-banthine, atropine and belladonna) to block the action of acetylcholine on the sweat glands often produces side effects such as dryness of the mouth, blurring of vision, dizziness, palpitation and urinary retention which are more troublesome than the hyperhidrosis itself. In cases in which there is an obvious emotional factor, tranquilizers or antihistaminics (e.g., Benadryl, Atarax and Vistaril), for their sedative properties, may occasionally be of some help. In general, systemic therapy for hyperhidrosis is disappointing.

Topical therapy may consist of simple foot soaks with tap water, saline or Burow's solution. Soaking for 20 to 30 minutes will usually inhibit sweating locally for up to several hours. Formalin soaks (5 to 10 percent aqueous formalin solution) are also helpful but may cause overdrying with fissuring and sensitization.

The use of a noncaking dusting powder will help reduce perspiration. These powders should be of a simple absorbent type and those containing numerous "medications" incorporated into the powder should be avoided, since at times irritant or allergic reactions may occur.

Local radiation therapy for hyperhidrosis should not be used because of the danger of late radiodermatitis. In extreme cases, when all other measures have failed, one may consider sympathectomy. The second, third, and fourth lumbar ganglia are resected. The operation is permanently effective and there are no late adverse effects on the skin itself.

In our experience the following set of directions has proved helpful in controlling mild to moderate hyperhidrosis:

1. Soak feet in Burow's solution (1:20), morning and evening.
2. Dry feet well.
3. Dust powder freely into shoes and hosiery.
4. Cotton hose or peds are preferable. Change twice daily, morning and evening.
5. Change shoes twice daily, morning and evening.

DYSHIDROSIS

Dyshidrosis, also called pompholyx, is a recurrent eruption of numerous deep-seated vesicles occurring singly and in groups on the palms and soles with minimal inflammatory signs. Hyperhidrosis frequently is also present. The name, dyshidrosis, is unfortunate since studies have failed to show that the primary lesion of dyshidrosis is a sweat retention vesicle. Rather dyshidrosis is an eczematous reaction pattern of the skin, unique by virtue of the anatomy of the affected sites. Secondary sweat retention may occur in the vesicles, with resulting exacerbation of the dyshidrosis.

Therapy for dyshidrosis is similar to that described for hyperhidrosis. In addition, topical steroids and systemic broad spectrum antibiotics are often useful therapeutic modalities.

BROMHIDROSIS

Bromhidrosis or foul-smelling sweat frequently occurs on the feet. Eccrine sweat itself, as secreted, is odorless. However, sweat promotes bacterial growth and the odor associated with sweating is the result of bacterial decomposition of surface protein debris.

Therapy should be directed toward the hyperhidrosis, as discussed previously, against the bacterial flora of the skin by the use of antibacterial soaps and against the proteinaceous debris by frequent washing.

ANHIDROSIS

Anhidrosis is the inability of the body to produce and/or deliver sweat to the skin surface. Anhidrosis of the feet may be part of a generalized anhidrosis or may be local. Causes of generalized anhidrosis are: damage to the hypothalamus such as in heatstroke, neurosurgical procedures, tumors, and mechanical trauma; hysteria; anticholinergic drugs; congenital ectodermal defect; Atabrine dermatitis; skin conditions such as atopic dermatitis, contact dermatitis, pemphigus, exfoliative dermatitis; hormonal disturbances such as Addison's disease, myxedema, diabetes mellitus and diabetes insipidus; poisoning as by arsenic, fluorine, formaldehyde, lead, morphine and thallium; fluid imbalance; malignancy; glomerulonephritis; and cirrhosis.

Causes of anhidrosis localized in the feet may be cord lesions as with poliomyelitis, multiple sclerosis, syringomyelia and tumors; alcoholic polyneuritis; leprosy; nerve tumors; diabetes mellitus; gout; orthostatic hypotension; localized congenital absence of sweat glands; atrophy of glands due to senile skin, radiodermatitis, lymphedema, acrodermatitis chronica atrophicans, etc; antiperspirants; interference with blood supply in skin as by continuous pressure of a cast; and skin diseases such as lichen planus and psoriasis.

Therapy must be directed toward the responsible etiologic agent.

11

Heritable Diseases

An extraordinary variety of heritable syndromes upon occasion may involve the skin or nails of the feet. However, as we have done in other sections of this text, we have selected certain of the disorders to present here.

PALMOPLANTAR KERATODERMAS

The palmoplantar keratodermas are a group of hereditary disorders characterized by diffuse or focal thickening of the soles and palms, or occasionally, of only one of these sites.

The six following syndromes are all characterized by an autosomal dominant inheritance pattern:

1. **Diffuse Palmoplantar Keratoderma (Tylosis; Thost-Unna syndrome).** In this disorder a diffuse thickening of the palms and soles is noted in early infancy and is often fully developed by the age of 6 months. The hyperkeratosis is smooth, uniform and sharply demarcated from normal skin by an erythematous border. Hyperhidrosis and painful fissuring may occur, but some patients are asymptomatic. The nails may be normal or thickened.

An association between esophageal carcinoma and palmoplantar keratoderma has been reported in several families. In these cases the hyperkeratosis did not appear in infancy but rather between the ages of 5 and 15 years.

The hyperkeratosis will frequently respond strikingly to topical vitamin A acid 0.3 percent in petrolatum as reported by Heiss and Gross.[1]

2. **Mutilating Keratoderma (Vohwinkel syndrome).** In this disorder the keratoderma of the palms and soles appears in infancy and shows a surface honeycombed with small depressions. Linear keratoses and starfish-shaped keratoses have been noted on the knees, elbows and the dorsal aspects of the hands and feet. At any time after age 5 constrictive bands develop around the smaller digits and progress to auto amputation of the affected digits.

3. **Progressive Palmoplantar Keratoderma (Greither's syndrome).** This rare syndrome also begins in infancy, but unlike tylosis is characterized by slow progression over a variable number of years, sometimes until the fourth decade. The sides and dorsa of the feet and hands as well as irregular patches on the legs and arms may be affected with patchy hyperkeratotic lesions.

4. **Punctate Keratoderma.** This genodermatosis is marked by punctate, round to oval, hard keratotic lesions on the palms and soles, and develops between 15 and 30 years of age. The keratotic plugs may be removed by trauma and leave a depression surrounded by a horny wall. Onychogryphosis, longitudinal fissuring of the nails and other nail dystrophies may occur in association. Arsenical keratoses may simulate this keratoderma.

5. **Striate Keratoderma.** In this syndrome linear keratoses involving the soles or palms may extend onto the digits.

6. **Disseminate Palmoplantar Keratoderma With Corneal Dystrophy.** This hyperkeratotic syndrome is manifested by diffuse, punctate or linear keratoderma which may be associated with corneal dystrophy or comma-shaped, punctate or dendritic opacities. The keratoderma does not develop until the second decade of life.

The following three disorders are characterized by an autosomal recessive inheritance pattern:

1. **Mal de Meleda.** This rare syndrome, named after the Dalmatian island of Meleda (Mljet) is primarily due to inbreeding. Redness of the palms and soles in early infancy is followed by scaling and thickening which is more often diffuse than focal. The sides and dorsa of the feet and hands are covered in part by the hyperkeratotic lesions. Hyperhidrosis, with secondary eczematization is common. Circumscribed areas on the knuckles, knees and elbows may be affected as well. A sharp erythematous border surrounds the lesions. The area of involvement tends to increase with age.

2. **Palmoplantar Keratoderma with Periodontosis (Papillon-Lefevre syndrome).** This rare syndrome exhibits redness and thickening of the palms and soles beginning at ages 1 to 5 years and extending along the Achilles tendon and the sides of the hands and feet. Hyperhidrosis and periodontosis are present. The latter causes loss of deciduous and permanent teeth early in life.

3. **Circumscribed Palmoplantar Keratoderma.** This keratoderma develops as tender callosities at pressure points on the soles and palms. Mental deficiency, leukoplakia of the buccal mucous membrane and corneal dystrophies may be associated.

ICHTHYOSIFORM DERMATOSES

The classification adapted for this group of disorders is largely that of Frost and Van Scott,[2] based upon epidermal proliferation rates, histopathological findings and clinical characteristics.

1. **Ichthyosis Vulgaris.** Ichthyosis vulgaris is inherited as an autosomal dominant disorder, possibly with incomplete penetrance. It is not present at birth but begins between the ages of 1 to 4 years and becomes more severe over the next several years. Small, fine scales occur on the trunk and arms with larger scales noted on the legs. The antecubital and popliteal fossae are relatively spared. The turnover rate

of the skin is less than normal, that is, the horny layer is abnormally retained. The rate of keratinization is not increased.

2. **Lamellar Ichthyosis.** This disorder is inherited as an autosomal recessive trait although spontaneous mutations probably occur. Universal erythema and scaling from birth to adulthood is usual. The flexures are not spared. In an untreated case, the scales are large, thin, gray-brown in color, centrally adherent with an elevated margin. Ectropion and corneal scarring with vascularization occasionally occur.

3. **Epidermolytic Hyperkeratosis.** Present at birth as a thick scaly mantle, the skin is shed almost immediately to leave a raw body surface. Thick gray-brown often verrucous scales then form over most of the body, particularly in the flexural creases such as the antecubital and popliteal fossae. Flaccid bullae due to bacterial infection of the skin may occur. The inheritance is autosomal dominant.

4. **X-Linked Ichthyosis.**[3] Generalized dry skin and scaling, particularly of the legs, arms, trunk and neck occur in very early infancy in this sex-linked dermatosis. The characteristic scales are large and yellow, brown or black in color. Palms and soles are uninvolved. Deep corneal opacities are noted not only in affected individuals, but also in the carriers of this trait. They are of no clinical significance but are useful in determining the type of ichthyosis. An association with mental retardation, skeletal anomalies and pituitary hypogonadism has been reported.

5. **Psoriasiform Erythroderma.** These patients show generalized erythema and scaling, often from infancy. The scales are micaceous and desquamate in large quantities. Clinically and histologically the disorder is identical to generalized psoriasis. This disorder is not an ichthyosis but is included here, since it is often confused clinically with the ichthyotic states.

Histologic studies are helpful in differentiating the clinical types of ichthyosis.

Therapy for all types of ichthyosis consists of hydration baths followed by the application of hydrophilic ointment, aqua and aquaphor or petrolatum or by applying 40 percent urea in Keri lotion; 3 percent salicylic acid added to the emollients may also be helpful. Antibacterial soaps and systemic antibiotics will heal the bullae and eradicate the odor of epidermolytic hyperkeratosis.

EPIDERMOLYSIS BULLOSA

This is a group of genetically determined syndromes characterized by bulla formation as a response to trauma.

1. **Epidermolysis Bullosa Simplex.** This is an autosomal dominant disorder usually first manifested, when the infant begins to crawl or walk, by clear tense bullae on the palms, soles and knees or other areas of frequent trauma. The lesions heal without scarring. Some patients may improve at puberty, but in any case, longevity is not impaired.

2. **Cockayne Syndrome or Recurrent Bullous Eruption of the Feet.** This disorder, also referred to as the "march syndrome," is variously considered as a mild variant of the simplex form of epidermolysis bullosa or as a separate entity. Bullae develop on the feet subsequent to friction as in prolonged marches in the army, or subsequent to normal trauma of walking, especially during the summer months. Affected individuals seldom have blisters on parts other than their feet.

3. **Hyperplastic Epidermolysis Bullosa.** In this autosomal dominant disorder bullae develop on the knees and feet, forehead and hands as well as on other sites of trauma either in infancy or not until puberty or later. They heal with atrophic scars and milia or at times keloids. Ichthyosis, keratosis pilaris and palmoplantar keratoderma with hyperhidrosis and thickened dystrophic nails are common. Leukoplakia of the buccal mucosa may develop following repeated erosions at the site.

4. **Polydysplastic Epidermolysis Bullosa.** This form of epidermolysis bullosa is inherited as an autosomal recessive trait. Bullae appear at birth or in early infancy. Bullae develop on the feet and legs as well as in any traumatized area of the body. The bullae are large, flaccid and may be hemorrhagic. Scarring with pseudowebbing of the digits is common following repeated injury. Squamous cell carcinoma may develop on the legs in scarred atrophic skin. Scarring of the conjunctiva, mucous membranes and esophagus may also occur. Leukoplakia of the buccal mucosa with subsequent carcinoma formation, stricture of the esophagus leading to aspiration pneumonitis and occasionally to carcinoma of the esophagus have been reported.

5. **Epidermolysis Bullosa Letalis.** This autosomal recessive disorder is usually incompatible with life. Bullae develop within hours after birth leading to the shedding of sheets of skin. The mucous membranes are extensively involved. The entire picture presents an insuperable nursing problem and most children do not survive 3 months.

POROKERATOSIS

1. **Porokeratosis of Mibelli.** This is a benign disorder of keratinization characterized by extending plaques of hyperkeratosis followed by atrophy. The original lesion, a horny papule, gradually enlarges to form a plaque of circinate or irregular contour. The periphery of the plaques is raised, and from this raised area, a thin crest of keratin emerges. The central zone of the plaque may be normal or atrophic. The feet, hands, face and upper trunk are often affected. Most cases begin in childhood. A dominant inheritance pattern is occasionally manifested, but many random cases occur.

2. **Disseminated Superficial Actinic Porokeratosis.** In this autosomal dominant disorder described by Chernosky and Freeman,[4] follicular keratotic papules which evolve to annular keratotic lesions occur primarily on sun exposed sites such as the face, legs and arms. The lesions tend to enlarge slowly in an irregular circinate fashion. The eruption tends to regress during the winter months and exacerbate in

the summer. Symptomatic complaints such as pruritus are minimal. Clinically the lesions differ from those of porokeratosis of Mibelli but the histologic picture is the same though the findings are minimal.

ANHIDROTIC ECTODERMAL DYSPLASIA

This disorder is recessive in inheritance and 90 percent of the cases are males. Partial or complete absence of sweat glands and other epidermal appendages results in absent or reduced sweating, hypotrichosis and total or partial anodontia. The manifestations of the syndrome are widely variable. In the complete form there is a characteristic facies with prominent chin and frontal ridges, saddle nose, thick everted lips, large ears and sparse hair. The skin is dry and smooth, with fine wrinkles leading to an appearance of premature aging. When the ability to produce sweat is markedly reduced, exertion or a hot environment may cause the individual to become very uncomfortable.

There is no available satisfactory therapy.

DYSKERATOSIS CONGENITA

This syndrome consists of nail dystrophy, atrophy and pigmentation of the skin and leukoplakia. It is inherited as a partially sex-linked recessive disorder with almost all cases occurring in males.

The nail changes usually appear first with the nails becoming dystrophic and being shed between the ages of 5 and 13 years.

Reticulated brownish pigmentation along with some atrophy and telangiectasia results in a poikilodermatous appearance of the skin. These changes usually begin 2 or 3 years after the nail changes and reach their maximum within 5 years. The changes are most prominent on the neck and thighs but also involve large areas of the trunk.

The skin over the dorsa of the hands and feet is atrophic, shiny and transparent. Thickening and hyperhidrosis of the palms and soles may also occur.

The mucous membrane involvement consists of leukoplakia and is significant because of a high risk of carcinoma occurring in the areas of leukoplakia.

Many cases have shown an associated blood dyscrasia, with the precise type varying.

The prognosis is rather poor with a fatal outcome due to either a carcinoma or the blood dyscrasia.

PACHYONYCHIA CONGENITA

In this autosomal dominantly inherited disorder, the finger- and toenails develop a yellow thickening and curvature which may be present at birth or occur progressively over the first 5 years of life. Repeated infection and swelling of the nail folds and repeated shedding of the nails often occur. Subungual hyperkeratosis may be severe.

Keratoderma and hyperhidrosis of the palms and soles become apparent during childhood.

Leukoplakia of the tongue, buccal mucosa and larynx is very common during the teen-age years and may undergo malignant changes.

No treatment is available.

DARIER'S DISEASE (Keratosis follicularis)

Darier's disease, a disease of unknown etiology, is inherited as an autosomal dominant but most pedigrees do not extend beyond two generations because the marriage rate and fertility are low.

The distinctive lesion is a greasy crusted papule which may be flesh-colored or yellow-brown. Warty or papillomatous masses result from the coalescence of lesions and may be malodorous. The lesions most commonly occur on the chest, upper back and shoulders, lumbosacral and buttocks areas, scalp, face and the flexures. When the papules occur on the dorsal surfaces of the hands or feet, they resemble flat warts or acrokeratosis verruciformis. Punctate keratoses or minute pits are seen on the palms and soles. Keratoderma of the palms and soles is seen in approximately 10 percent of cases.

TUBEROUS SCLEROSIS

The characteristic features of this syndrome are epilepsy, mental retardation and skin lesions.

Epilepsy develops in about 80 percent of the cases and usually appears in infancy or early childhood, thus often antedating the appearance of the skin lesions by years.

Mental deficiency is noted in about 70 percent of cases and may be progressive.

The characteristic skin manifestations are: (1) adenoma sebaceum of Pringle, which are yellowish or telangiectatic firm papules occurring on the nasolabial folds, cheeks and chin; (2) the shagreen patch which is a thickened plaque located in the lumbosacral area; and (3) the periungual fibromata occurring on either the finger- or toenails at or after puberty. The fibromas appear as firm, smooth, flesh-colored tumors protruding from under the nail folds.

References

1. Heiss, H.B., and Gross, P.R.: Keratosis palmaris et plantaris treatment with topically applied vitamin A acid. Arch. Derm., *101*:100, 1970.

2. Frost, P., and Van Scott, E.J.: Ichthyosiform dermatoses. Arch. Derm., *94*:113, 1966.

3. Wells, R.S., and Kerr, C.B.: Clinical features of autosomal dominant and sex-linked ichthyosis in an English population. Brit. Med. J., *1*:947, Apr. 16, 1966.

4. Chernosky, M.E., and Freeman, R.G.: Disseminated superficial actinic porokeratosis (DSAP). Arch. Derm., *96*:611, 1967.

12

Miscellaneous Disorders

INGROWN TOENAILS

The so-called ingrown toenail may be a simple incurved nail or a true ingrown nail. While there are similarities in the treatment of each, significant differences do exist.

In the simple incurved nail (Fig. 12-1), the lateral aspects of the nail are markedly curved inward resulting in tenderness and pain. Therapy consists of packing cotton or lamb's wool under the advancing edge of the curved nail, thereby forcing it upward sufficiently to allow the nail to grow over the skin of the toe rather than into it. The packing is kept in place for the several months required. Prophylactic therapy consists of cutting the nails straight across and not too short.

In a true ingrown toenail, a pointed spicule of nail, that remains attached to the lateral portion of the nail following improper trimming, penetrates into the soft tissues of the toe as the nail plate grows forward (Fig. 12-2). This results in exquisite pain and often secondary infection.

Therapy consists of locating the nail sliver and removing it by cutting it away with a straight-edge nail cutting forceps followed by treating the infection with warm soaks and antibiotics, topical and systemic. When the infection has cleared, packing is placed under the nail as described previously for the incurved nail and the nail plate is allowed to grow out over it.

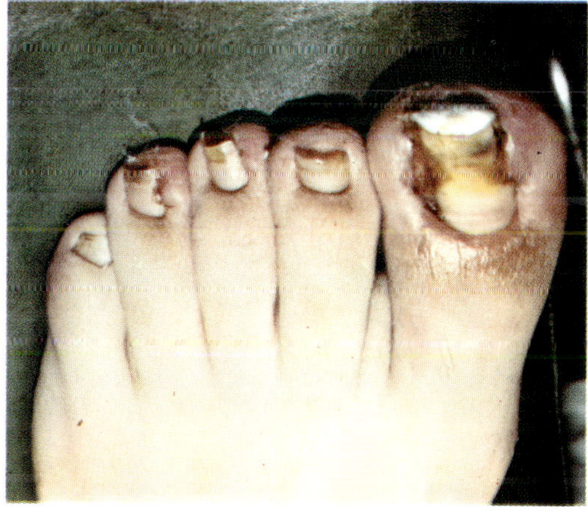

Fig. 12-1. Ingrown toenails.

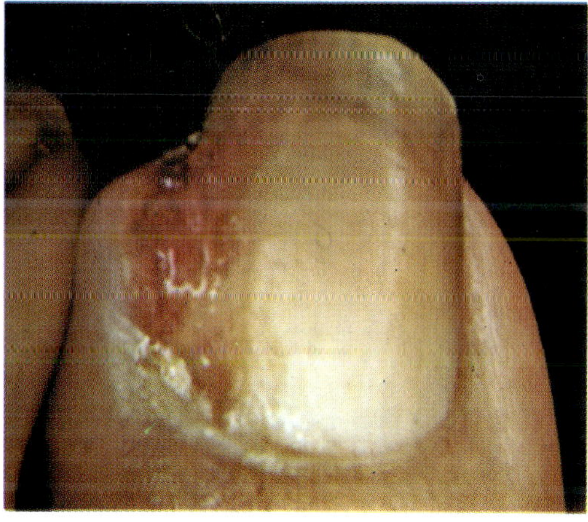

Fig. 12-2. Ingrown toenail.

PIEZOGENIC PAPULES

This disorder is not uncommon, though often unrecognized. Herniation of fatty subcutaneous tissue, through a defect of the connective tissue into the dermis, produces lesions which are not noted when the patient is recumbent but become apparent when the upright position is assumed. The most common site is the sides of the heels. The patient is asymptomatic when reclining; the herniations may remain asymptomatic or become painful when the patient stands.[1,2]

Palliative measures, such as supportive devices in the shoes and a change from a standing occupation to one of a more sedentary nature, are helpful. In some instances, surgical correction, excision of the fatty tissue protrusion at its base, may be indicated.

References

1. Shelley, W. B., and Rawnsley, H. M.: Painful feet due to herniation of fat. JAMA, *205*:308, 1968.
2. Galinski, A.W.: Cutaneous herniations. A case report. J. Am. Podiat. Ass. *60*:128,1970.

PURPLE TOES

Recently Bamshad and Dickhaus[1] reported an interesting complication of anticoagulant therapy. Their patient developed a deep purple discoloration of the toes, soles and dorsal aspect of the feet one week after the institution of Coumadin therapy. When Coumadin was discontinued and a non-coumarin type anticoagulant was substituted, the discoloration gradually disappeared. Petechiae, stasis dermatitis and edema, which had been present previously, remained after the resolution of the purple discoloration. The mechanism responsible was thought to be an unusual vasodilatory effect of the coumarin type drug.

References

1. Bamshad, J., and Dickhaus, D.W.: Purple toes. Cutis, *6*:639, 1970.

ECCRINE POROMA

The eccrine poroma was first described by Pinkus *et al.* in 1956.[1] It is a benign growth which is considered by most authors to originate from the distal and intra-epidermal portion of the eccrine sweat duct,[2,3,4] though this concept has not been universally accepted by all authors.

The lesion is a nontender, reddish, soft tumor which protrudes from a shallow cuplike invagination (Fig. 12-3). The tumor occurs mainly on the palm or sole and rarely is seen on the head, trunk and extremities. Poromas are usually single but Goldner[5] has reported a case in which there were more than 100 such tumors on the palms and soles. Most lesions appear in persons over the age of 40 years and there is no sex predilection.[6,7] Histologically the lesion is quite characteristic but has been occasionally mistakenly diagnosed as a basal cell epithelioma.

The lesions are benign and conservative surgical excision is curative, but recurrences will occur after a shave biopsy.[8]

References

1. Pinkus, H., Rogin, J.R., and Goldman, P.: Eccrine poroma. Arch. Derm., *74*:511, 1956.

2. Hashimoto, K., and Lever, W.F.: Eccrine poroma. J. Invest. Derm., *43*:237, 1964.

3. Sanderson, K.V., and Ryan, E.A.: The histochemistry of eccrine poroma. Brit. J. Derm., *75*:86, 1963.

4. Holubar, K., and Wolff, K.: Intra-epidermal eccrine poroma. Cancer, *23*:626, 1969.

5. Goldner, R.: Eccrine poromatosis. Arch. Derm., *101*:606, 1970.

6. Hyman, A.B., and Brownstein, M.H.: Eccrine poroma. Dermatologica, *138*:29, 1969.

7. Hashimoto, K., and Lever, W.F.: Appendage Tumors of the Skin. Springfield. (Ill.), Charles C Thomas, 1968.

8. Morris, J., Wood, M.G., and Samitz, M.H.: Eccrine poroma. Arch. Derm., *98*:162, 1968.

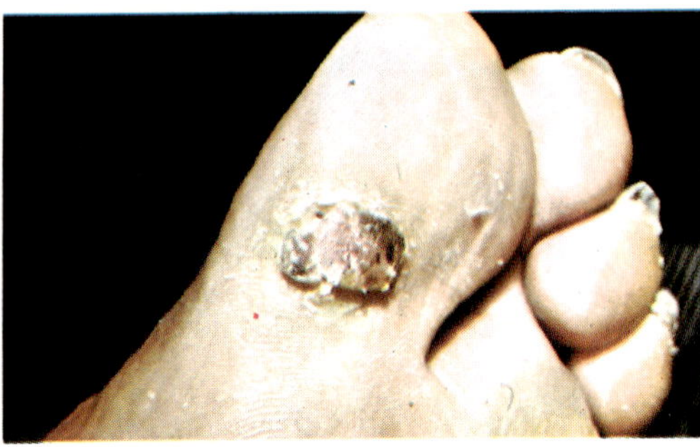

Fig. 12-3. Eccrine poroma—sharp demarcation of protruding tumor from surrounding tissue.

ELEPHANTIASIS NOSTRA VERRUCOSA (Lymphostasis verruciformis)

Elephantiasis is characterized by enlargement and deformity of the involved area, usually a limb. These changes are due to hypertrophic fibrosis of the skin and subcutaneous tissues resulting from blocking of the lymphatics.

Elephantiasis is of various types:

1. Congenital (Milroy's disease): congenital and familial form
2. Tropical (filaria, *F. bancrofti)*
3. Nostra of the temperate zone
4. Symptomatic or pseudoelephantiasis secondary to syphilis, frambesia, mycoses, neoplasms, surgery.

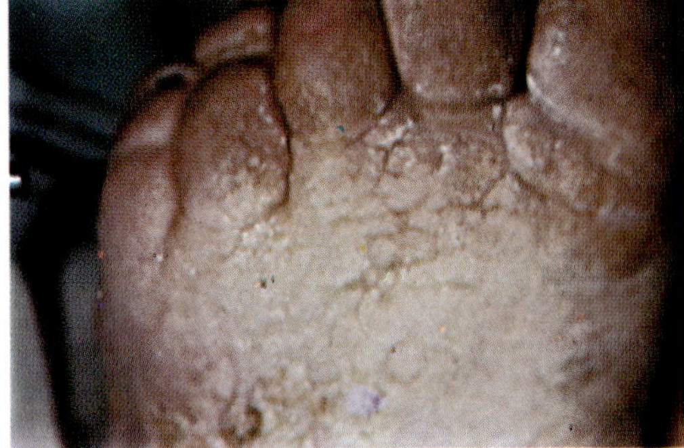

Fig. 12-5. Lymphostasis verruciformis. Close-up of lesions on toes.

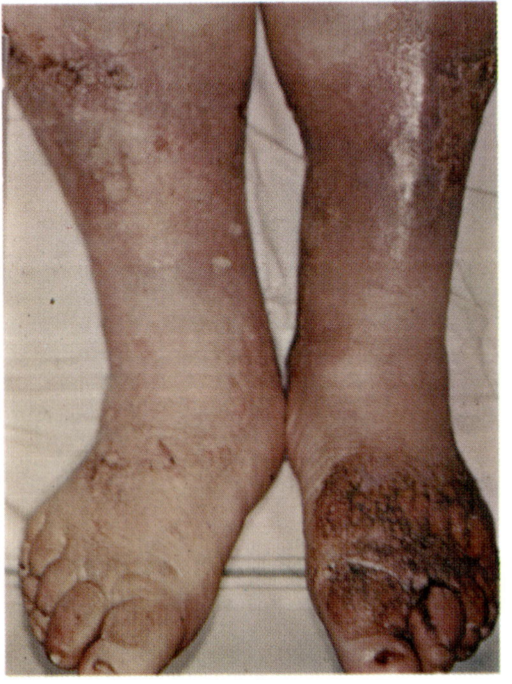

Fig. 12-4. Lymphostasis verruciformis.

Some individuals show a distinct tendency to experience recurrent episodes of erysipelas and cellulitis of the lower leg, ankles and toes. An elevated temperature and pain in the inguinal region usually accompany an attack. Frequently insignificant trauma is the precipitating factor. After numerous attacks, occurring over a period of time in the same area, permanent, firm brawny edema with hypertrophic warty epidermal changes of the skin appear in the involved portions of the extremity, leading to elephantiasis nostra verrucosa (Figs. 12-4, 12-5).

In lymphostasis verruciformis, chronic low-grade pyoderma is often present, though frequently it is not clinically apparent. Poor hygiene is a contributing factor.

Prophylaxis is the most important aspect of therapy but when the changes are established, long-term low-dose antibiotic therapy and the wearing of a pressure gradient stocking are helpful. Forty percent urea lotion or cream will reduce marked hyperkeratotic debris.

KERATODERMA PLANTARIS (Acquired)

Keratoderma plantaris may be acquired as well as hereditary. Numerous inflammatory disorders, such as psoriasis, lichen planus, syphilis, chronic arsenic intoxication and Reiter's disease may give rise to hyperkeratosis of the soles. Palmar and plantar keratoderma have been described in association with systemic cancers; however, this relationship has not been established with certainty. Occasionally, patients are seen who have striking plantar hyperkeratosis for which no etiology is established and whose family history is negative for similar conditions.

Acquired hyperkeratosis of the soles has, in the past, been treated with macerating soaks or keratolytic agents such as salicylic acid, forms of treatment which have been messy, inconvenient and rather unsatisfactory.

Heiss and Gross[1] reported excellent success with the application of 0.3 percent vitamin A acid ointment twice daily with plastic occlusion during the night. This would appear to be an effective and relatively simple therapeutic approach to a previously difficult problem (Figs. 12-6, 12-7).

1. Heiss, H.B., and Gross, P.R.: Keratosis palmaris and plantaris treatment with topically applied vitamin A acid. Arch. Derm., *101*:100, 1970.

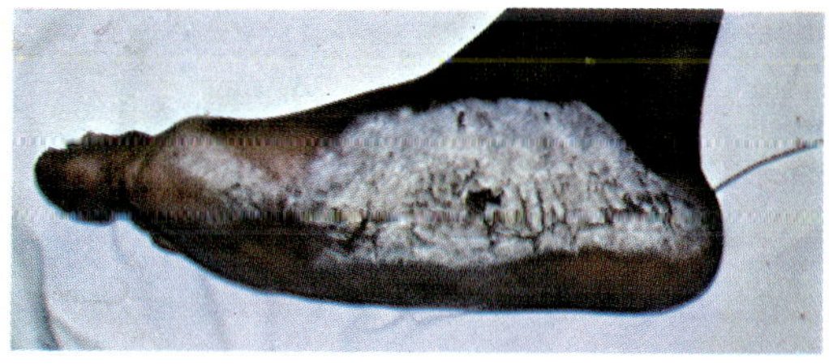

Fig. 12-6. Keratoderma plantaris (before treatment).

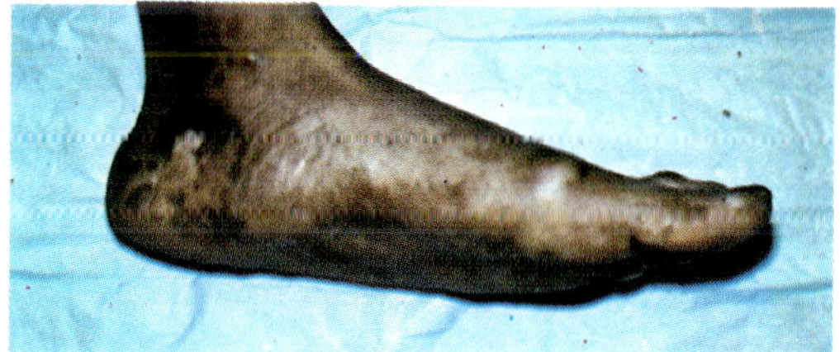

Fig. 12-7. Keratoderma plantaris following treating with 0.3 percent vitamin A acid under occlusion.

REITER'S DISEASE

Reiter's disease classically consists of urethritis, arthritis and conjunctivitis but is also often associated with lesions of both the skin and mucous membranes.

The etiology is unclear. Most cases are sporadic and usually follow sexual exposure; epidemics have occurred following dysentery. Various theories have attempted to implicate the gonococcus, Shigella and pleuropneumonia-like organisms or an autoimmune hypersensitivity phenomenon. More recently viruses of the Bedsonia group have been implicated and the accumulating evidence is fairly convincing. However, the mechanism of the complete Reiter's syndrome, as contrasted to the etiology of the urethritis, remains unknown.

Most cases occur in young adult males in whom urethritis is often the initial manifestation. The urethritis may vary from an acute, painful, hemorrhagic purulent drainage to a mild, often unnoticed, clear discharge. The remaining portions of the syndrome follow in approximately 10 to 14 days, though the mucocutaneous lesions may be delayed for 2 months or longer.

The conjunctivitis is noted in about 50 percent of cases, is usually bilateral, transient and rather mild. Of the various components of the syndrome it is the one most likely to be overlooked by history or on examination. Attacks usually last for 5 to 10 days, though occasionally they may be more prolonged. Recurrences of conjunctivitis tend to be unilateral.

Iritis has been reported in about 8 percent of initial attacks but in as many as 30 to 50 percent of recurrent protracted cases. Keratitis and ulceration of the cornea are rare. Interstitial keratitis, optic neuritis and glaucoma have been reported.

Arthritis is the dominant feature of the syndrome and occurs in at least 90 percent of cases. The joints are usually bilaterally and symmetrically involved with weight-bearing joints of the lower extremity and the sacro-iliac region the areas most frequently and severely affected. Initially the joint involvement is transient but recurrent attacks may lead to permanent deformity and may resemble ankylosing spondylitis. X-ray changes may be seen in up to 40 percent of patients but may also be absent, even in patients suffering repeated attacks.

Skin lesions consist of a marked keratoderma, usually of the soles but may involve other areas, and nail dystrophy. The keratoderma has in the past been termed keratoderma blennorrhagica but this term has been largely discarded since it implies a gonococcal etiology. The keratoderma occurs in about 8 percent of the venereal cases and less often in the postdysentery cases. It begins as a dull red macule which evolves to resemble a vesicle but the lesion remains hard. The center of the lesion changes to thicken and form massive cone-shaped hyperkeratotic masses, in some instances resembling rupial psoriasis. In moist, intertriginous areas cheesy, flaccid pustular lesions develop. Rarely widespread psoriasiform lesions may involve the entire body.

The nail involvement begins as an erythematous swelling of the posterior nail fold; subsequently the nails become grossly distorted by massive subungual hyperkeratosis and nail plate thickening and are shed. The skin lesions involute in from 8 weeks to 10 months.

Mucous membrane lesions occur in up to 50 percent of venereal cases and in about 10 percent of postdysentery cases. A circinate painless balanitis lasting a few days to several weeks and erythematous papules, opaque vesicles or shallow erosions of the oral mucosa are seen.

Thrombophlebitis associated with arthritis of the knee has been reported as have myocarditis, pericarditis, aortic incompetence, heart-block, pleurisy and pulmonary infiltrations.

The prognosis is generally good, since attacks are self-limiting, lasting a few weeks to several months. However, recurrences are not rare and may lead to disabling arthritis as well as, occasionally, to other complications mentioned previously.

The self-limiting nature of Reiter's disease makes therapy difficult to evaluate and should encourage the physician to be conservative in his therapeutic approaches. For the arthritic complaints, bed rest, salicylates, heat and occasionally a short course of phenylbutazone are effective. Broad spectrum antibiotics should be used for the urethritis. Cutaneous lesions usually respond to soaks, topical steroids and keratolytic agents. In severe cases systemic steroids or methotrexate have seemed helpful but their use should be reserved for only the most severe and recalcitrant cases.

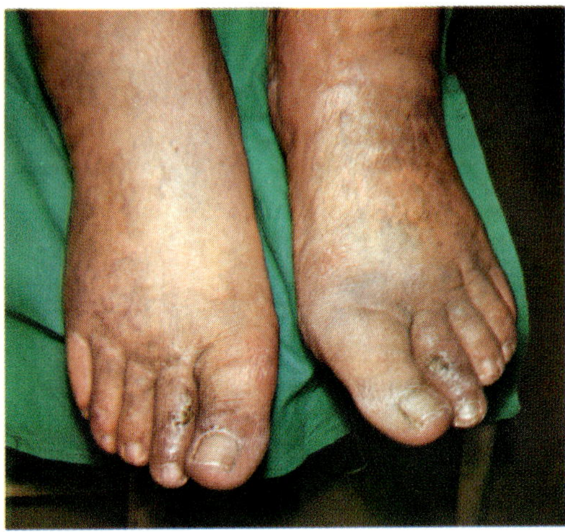

Fig. 12-8. Bilateral gout in great and second toes of woman. Past history of extensive venous disease and symptoms of pain with minimal erythema and swelling delayed correct diagnosis being made.

GOUT

Gout is an inborn error of metabolism which results in hyperuricemia, deposits of urates in articular cartilages and the skin, and attacks of an acute arthritis. Uric acid deposits give rise to tophi of the ears, bursae of the elbow and knees, in the tendons of the fingers, wrists, toes and ankles as well as to lumpy deposits in the skin over joints.

In classical acute attacks of gouty arthritis the great toe, ankle or foot is involved by a painful deep red, hot swelling which is tender to the touch. A bacterial cellulitis may be mistakenly diagnosed. Gouty attacks may also be misdiagnosed when they are not typical in location or symptomatology or occur in areas of preexisting disease (Fig. 12-8). Gouty attacks may follow minor local trauma, mild illnesses or other factors but often there is no precipitating cause. Serum uric acid levels are often elevated but need not be. Gout occurs primarily in males until age 40, after which a significant number of cases are women, though males still predominate.

An index of suspicion will lead to the correct diagnosis. Therapy consists of colchicine for acute attacks and probenecid for chronic gout.

Index

Numerals in *italics* indicate color illustrations.